Your book looks great....I think you did a great job simplifying the p understand and appreciate what goes on behind the scenes.

(Ben Robison, Chief Medical Physicist, Provision CARES Proton Therapy Center, Knoxville, Tennessee)

I am absolutely sold on proton treatment for prostate cancer treatment due to the cure rate, depending on the Gleason score, and absence of side effects. The availability of proton treatment needs more exposure.

(Glenn G. Butler, prostate cancer survivor treated with proton therapy)

Robert, thanks for your time and effort to make (proton therapy) better known. I received thirty-three fractions (treatments) with extreme satisfaction and encouragement.

(Jerald Ellington, prostate cancer survivor treated with proton therapy)

Thanks for your book. You've done a great service for a large number of people. Given the choice again, knowing what I know now, I still would choose proton therapy hands down, over any other form of prostate cancer treatment.

(John Wynd, prostate cancer survivor treated with proton therapy)

You did a very thorough job researching the information and an excellent work in writing about the proton process.

(Chuck Parmele, prostate cancer survivor treated with proton therapy)

I have been told your book is the best book on proton therapy on the market! Your book will help positively effect the lives of so many cancer patients, and I'm looking forward to sharing this with a lot of patients!

(Samantha Kirk, Patient Care Coordinator, Provision CARES Proton Therapy Center, Knoxville, Tennessee)

Robert Ferré's book "Best Prostate Cancer Treatment PROTON BEAM THERAPY" is a seminal work on Prostate Cancer treatment. Robert's book came to me at a most fortuitous time. I had just been diagnosed with prostate cancer and am now at that juncture where I must commit to a particular prostate cancer therapy. All males should read this book, especially if they are, like me, contemplating treatment advice being given by their Urological Oncologist for their already diagnosed prostate cancer or they suspect they should seek medical advice for a possible prostate problem.

George Davidson Greenly Jr., Former scientist at the Lawrence Livermore National Laboratory.

Facing the reality of aggressive cancer, few people would have the analytic calmness, tenacity, perseverance, and constructive assertiveness to keep calling, emailing, questioning, negotiating, compromising, and ultimately succeeding. This book is now, and will continue to be, enormously useful and comforting to countless cancer patients.

Jerry Stansell, retired Air Force officer

BEST PROSTATE CANCER TREATMENT: PROTON BEAM THERAPY

2018 UPDATE

ROBERT D. FERRÉ

Best Prostate Cancer Treatment: Proton Beam Therapy

Robert D. Ferré

First Edition: January, 2017
Updated Edition: August, 2018

ISBN: 978-1-940875-89-7

Labyrinth Enterprises, LLC

www.labyrinth-enterprises.com
San Antonio, Texas

Cover photo left: *A patient lies on the treatment table inside the gantry to receive proton beam therapy.*
Cover photo right: *The author and his wife Linda Ricketts celebrate Robert's post-treatment graduation ceremony by ringing the victory bell.*

TABLE OF CONTENTS

PROTON TECHNOLOGY

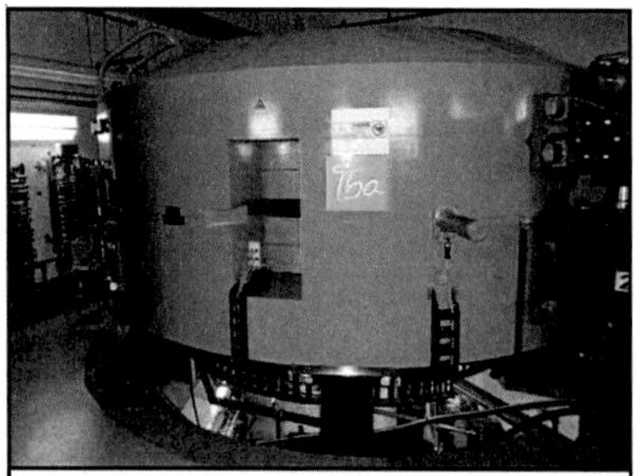

Cyclotron accelerates protons to two-thirds the speed of light

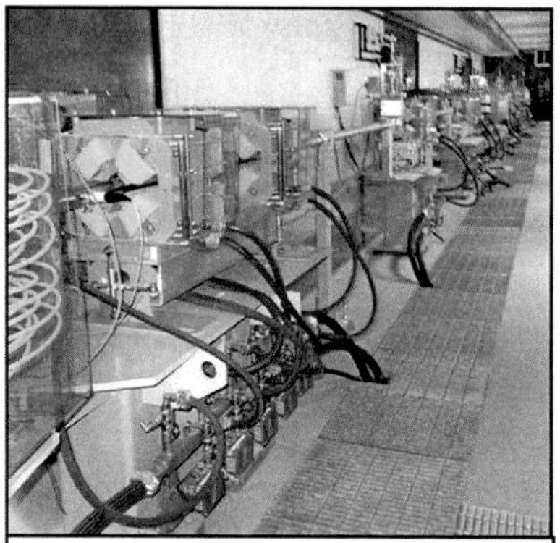

Magnets shape and control protons through beam line

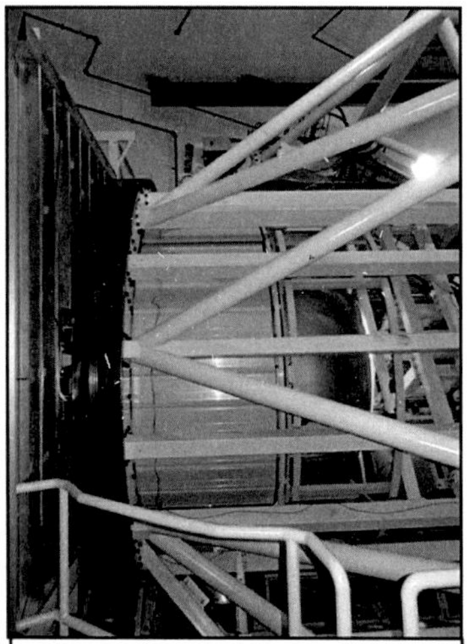

Huge gantry turns the beam a range of 360 degrees

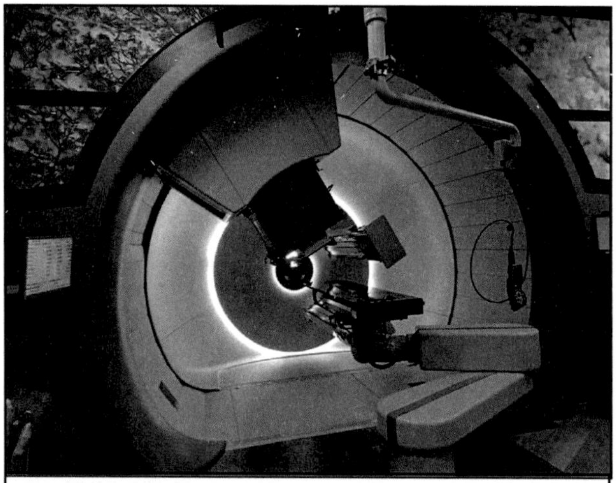

Beam reaches patient on highly adjustable treatment table

CHAPTER 1 PROSTATES AND PROTONS

This book describes proton therapy. Any man, spouse, relative, or friend of a man facing prostate cancer needs to read this book. It contains current information not available from any other single book.

A type of radiation treatment, proton therapy uses protons instead of X-rays to treat cancer. Because of their unique characteristics, protons (positively-charged hydrogen ions) successfully target the cancer while sparing the healthy tissue. I start with a quick summary, to be expanded upon later.

Protons (derived from hydrogen gas) are injected into a cyclotron which energizes them by accelerating them to two-thirds the speed of light. The subsequent beam of protons moves through a vacuum line controlled by magnets that organize, focus and direct the beam to the appropriate treatment room, where various devices shape, scatter, or scan the protons (depending on the system used), delivering them to the target where they release most of their energy in a big burst. Thereafter, the protons have no damaging exit through the body as do X-rays, a very critical distinction. Proton therapy comprises quite a story, which I tell in these pages, covering the following topics, among others:

- Why your urologist never mentions proton therapy.
- Proof that proton therapy gives the best result with the fewest side effects.
- How proton therapy outperforms X-ray radiation.
- The author's personal description of receiving proton therapy treatments.
- Recent technological advances in proton therapy not covered in older books.
- A special program that pays 80% of the cost of proton therapy for those on Medicare.
- How to deal with insurance companies and their resistance to proton therapy.
- The amazing physics of proton therapy and pencil beam scanning.
- The superiority of pencil beam scanning for other cancers besides prostate cancer.
- More than 150 full-color photos and illustrations.
- Obstacles and resistance to proton therapy.
- The future of proton therapy, compact equipment, lower prices, wider availability.
- Proton therapy centers currently in operation, and those planned or under construction.

This book recounts my experience receiving proton therapy for prostate cancer and explains the treatment itself, how it works, how to pay for it, who's doing it, and what the future holds. I don't cover any other forms of treatment, other than to compare them briefly to proton therapy.

IMPORTANT NOTICE

The purpose of this book is to give the reader information about proton therapy from my personal point of view as a previous patient treated with this technology. I am NOT giving medical advice. If you think you might want to have proton therapy, contact a proton center and ask for a consultation. Do NOT rely solely on the contents of this book. Seek proper medical advice from a source currently engaged in the application of proton therapy. You may contact me for corrections to this book or to elaborate on my personal experience, but NOT for medical advice, for which I am unqualified. I do, however, have very strong opinions, which I express freely in these pages. This is not a scientific report filled with footnotes and attributions. It's a personal account about the current state of proton therapy. If you disagree with me, feel free to write your own book.

In these pages I share not only the nature of proton therapy, but how and why it works. Therein lies the convincing evidence of its superiority as a cancer treatment. I have written a second book, entitled *Proton Therapy: Revolutionary Treatment for 80% of ALL Cancers*. It extends the information to a wide range of cancers, not just prostate. Both of my books are priced at one dollar above cost. My purpose is not personal enrichment, but spreading the word about proton therapy. I also have three websites pertaining to the subject:

www.ProtonTherapyBook.com
Here I include the photos and illustrations in my books plus additional information. You can learn much about proton therapy here without the need to even buy the books.

www.proton-beam-therapy.com
This is my blog site, in which I respond to current topics relevant to proton therapy. I also have links to newsletters and other links of interest.

www.proton-therapy-centers.com
This is an up-to-date list of proton therapy centers in the United States currently open for business, or in the planning or construction stages.

When prostate cancer took over my life, I studied every treatment option, including first person accounts of proton therapy. I find that those accounts differ in important ways from my experience in the fall of 2016. For example, technology vastly improved with the introduction of pencil beam scanning, hydrogel, and refined procedures. This gives relevance for this updated description to anyone investigating prostate cancer treatment.

The entire story of proton therapy and its medical application fascinates me: the foundational theory by a scientist apologetic for developing nuclear weapons, the heroic beginnings, and the current efforts to increase efficiency while reducing cost. I have no doubt that proton therapy represents the treatment of the present as well as the future.

I'd like to see this book in the waiting room of every urologist's office, but that's not very likely. Many urologists are surgeons. They have confidence in their skills and recommend surgery to virtually all their qualified patients. Unfortunately for surgeons, the same patients are the best candidates for proton therapy. In my estimation, as proton therapy increases in popularity, surgery will decrease considerably. It is not unusual for a new technology to have a negative impact on the older technology that it is replacing. Many (not all) urologists would like to keep proton therapy a secret.

Many men, shocked by their cancer diagnosis, immediately go for surgery to "get rid of it." Surgeons call surgery the most definitive solution, sure to eradicate the cancer. Yet in a surprising number of cases (23%), some cancer gets missed and requires additional treatment. It is not the gold standard it is claimed to be.

Having interviewed and questioned many men receiving proton therapy for prostate cancer, I asked if they were referred by their urologist. To a man they said no, without a single exception. They were advised to have surgery or X-rays. To protect their territory (unethically in my opinion) urologists fail to even mention proton therapy to their patients. Or if they do, they deem it unproven, experimental, no better than X-rays, unavailable, or far too expensive. Insurance companies tend to have the same opinion. In these pages I will counter these inaccuracies, misunderstandings, and false criticism.

X-ray radiologists find themselves in a similar fix. Early on, the question was whether protons were as effective as X-rays. Now the tables are turned, and radiologists are scrambling to show that X-rays are as effective as protons. Although categorized as a type of radiation, proton therapy uses charged particles (protons) rather than electromagnetic energy (X-rays). An enormous difference exists between the two, their capabilities, and how they function.

Typically, men receiving proton therapy must find their own way; this calls for motivation, courage, and determination. I was told that eighty-five percent of the patients where I was treated are self-referred. One man to whom I spoke was livid, telling me how his urologist had recommended an older, damaging form of X-rays; yet when the urologist was subsequently diagnosed with prostate cancer, he went to Jacksonville, Florida, to receive proton therapy! Another urologist gave the patient a booklet with seven potential treatment modalities, saying he should decide which one was best for him. Proton therapy was not included in the booklet.

When I asked my urologist about proton therapy, he shrugged and said, "We don't do that here." He's part of a large urological practice with twenty-six doctors and several locations. They're doing just fine without proton therapy, thank you very much.

I don't mean to vilify urologists and radiologists. They work to keep us healthy and functioning. Yet, they find themselves in a bind. If they sent everyone away for proton therapy, much of their livelihood would vanish.

Nor are protons the best choice for everyone. Treatment may involve travel to a distant proton center, require two months away from home and work, incur considerable expense, and lead to battling with insurance carriers.

Nor are there enough centers, yet, to handle the demand that would result from mass referrals. Those lucky enough to live near a proton therapy center often continue to go to their day jobs as usual, swinging by for their treatment before or after working hours.

Urologists should rejoice over the effectiveness of proton therapy. As astounding as it may sound, there are *no* urologists at the center which treated me (Provision CARES Proton Therapy Center in Knoxville, Tennessee), only oncologists and medical physicists. I'd never had a medical physicist before.

Like many other authors of books about prostate cancer, I want to rent billboards or take out television ads that say to men in the throes of decision: STOP! Don't blindly accept surgery or X-rays. You may have better choices. In Knoxville, Provision runs television ads that tactfully suggest to anyone diagnosed with cancer that they would be prudent to get a second opinion, which Provision offers.

I dedicate this book to all men facing the decision that I and legions of other men have had to make. I also gratefully acknowledge the love and support provided by my wife Linda throughout my cancer journey and my life. Without her, finding my way would have been much more difficult.

CHAPTER 2 THE FUTURE HAS ARRIVED

Here I give a quick overview of proton therapy and compare it to standard X-rays. In other chapters I cover in greater detail the physics of charged particles and dosimetry, the means by which one receives the most efficacious and accurate dose of cancer-killing protons.

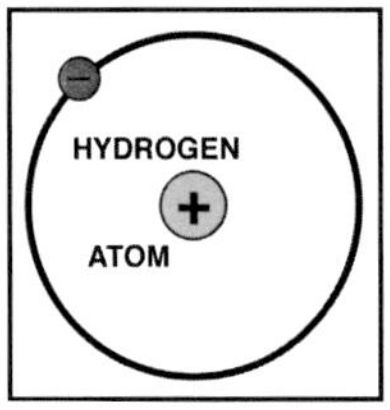

Even though they are quite dissimilar in how they perform, protons and X-rays are both classified as radiation therapy. Protons are derived from the nucleus of hydrogen atoms. X-rays are produced by electrons. The words can be a little confusing between X-rays (pHotons) and positively charged particles (pRotons), just one letter difference.

X-rays irradiate healthy tissue both before and after hitting the target. Protons, on the other hand, spare most of the healthy tissue. Because they have mass, protons have a unique quality which underlies the basis of their use for medical purposes. Protons don't keep going, like X-rays. Rather, they go a certain distance—depending on their speed, energy, and the medium in which they are traveling—and then release most of their energy in a big burst, after which they no longer exist. As a result, protons have no exit path as with X-rays.

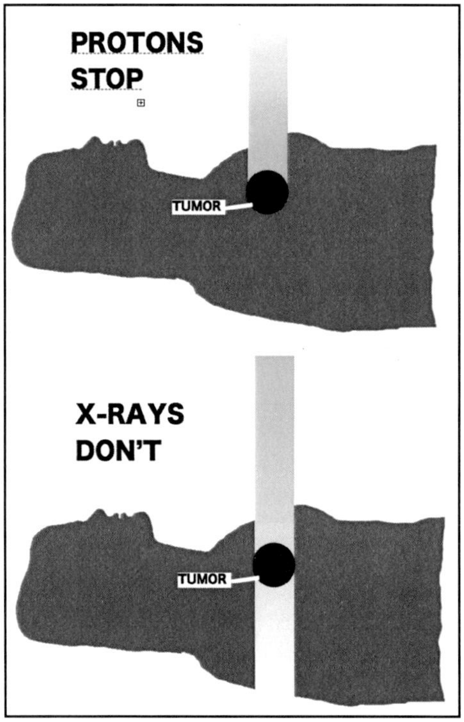

For treatment purposes, physicists can calculate the distance that protons travel so they can release their burst of energy within the intended target. I say target rather than prostate, because my target also included the seminal vesicles and lymph nodes. Producing, directing, and controlling protons takes enormously complex computations, equipment and well-trained people, hence the high cost. Happily, this cost continues to decrease as the technology matures and miniaturizes.

> *A proton and an X-ray stop at a bar on the way home from the cyclotron. After a couple of drinks, the bartender comes around and asks if they want another round. The X-ray says, "Sure, let's keep going." The proton says, "No thanks. I know when to stop."*

Insurance companies take the stand that surgery and both forms of radiation have equal results. Therefore, they won't cover proton therapy (which saves them a considerable amount of money).

While it's true that surgery, X-rays or protons all kill cancer, the difference in side effects can sometimes be downright scary.

For any modality, the possibility of secondary cancer or reoccurrence raises its ugly head. Proton therapy is by nature less invasive than surgery and causes less morbidity (damage to healthy tissue) than X-rays. This advantage escapes typical insurance companies which don't care if you wear diapers the rest of your life, or never have sex again, or have permanent bowel problems. Later, a whole chapter covers insurance issues (page 98).

When my prospective surgeon said he was going to "go wide" and "take out everything," I envisioned the prostate as this concise little walnut-size thing, with vine-like nerves embracing it and maybe a little margin around it. After seeing the size of the area necessary to treat the seminal vesicles and lymph nodes (see page 71), I was aghast at the considerable destruction surgery would have inflicted on my body, even if done precisely and robotically.

We should compare protons therapy to intensity modulated radiation therapy (IMRT) or other newer developments for X-rays. This definition of IMRT comes from the internet.

Intensity modulated radiation therapy is an advanced mode of high-precision radiotherapy that utilizes computer-controlled X-ray accelerators to deliver precise radiation doses to malignant tumors or specific areas within the tumors. The radiation dose is designed to conform to the three dimensional (3-D) shape of the tumor by modulating or controlling the intensity of the radiation beam to focus a higher radiation dose to the tumor while minimizing radiation exposure to surrounding normal tissue. (See: https://www.radiologyinfo.org/en/info.cfm?pg=imrt)

Notice their emphasis on precision. We will address that issue shortly. We will also see that X-rays are not three-dimensional, but protons are. All treatments have the goal expressed here, to maximize dose, get the most accurate results, and minimize damage to healthy tissue.

IMRT minimizes morbidity by using numerous rays of a smaller dose directed from around the target so that healthy tissue gets a lower dose while the target gets the total accumulated dose. Some types of X-rays send rays from all 360 degrees around the target, bathing virtually the entire area in radiation of one energy or another.

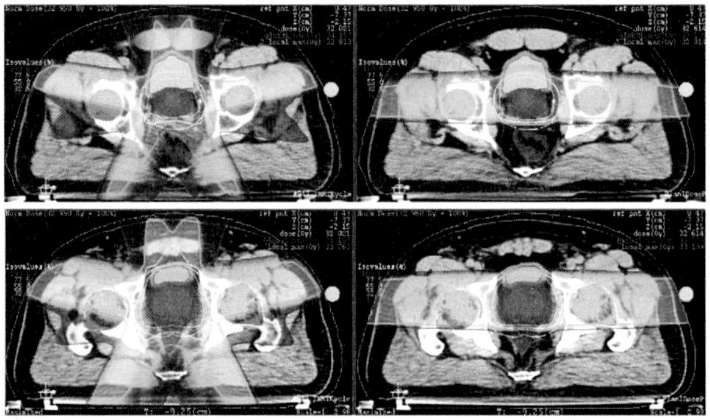

Prostate IMRT (left) IMPT @ 5% isodose

In the illustration, note how much more radiation healthy tissues receive with IMRT on the left than proton therapy on the right. Perhaps it doesn't matter to irradiate all of that tissue, but why chance it? This illustration was provided by the proton therapy center in Prague, The Czech Republic.

Proton therapy does expose some healthy tissue. During my treatment, the urethra within the prostate took a full-strength dose of protons. I was assured that fairly quickly this tissue heals itself, whereas the cancer doesn't. I received five treatments per week with weekends off. Spreading out the treatments allows this healing to take place in surrounding tissue by keeping swelling at a minimum. They could give the entire dose in one session and effectively destroy the cancer, but there would be extensive and unacceptable peripheral damage.

Cancer cells are more unstable than healthy ones. The protons damage and destabilize the DNA through a process of ionization (stealing their electrons), from which the cancer doesn't fully recover. With each session, the cancer recovers less and less, until it reaches a level from which it cannot recover or reproduce. The healthy tissue, on the other hand, returns to normal.

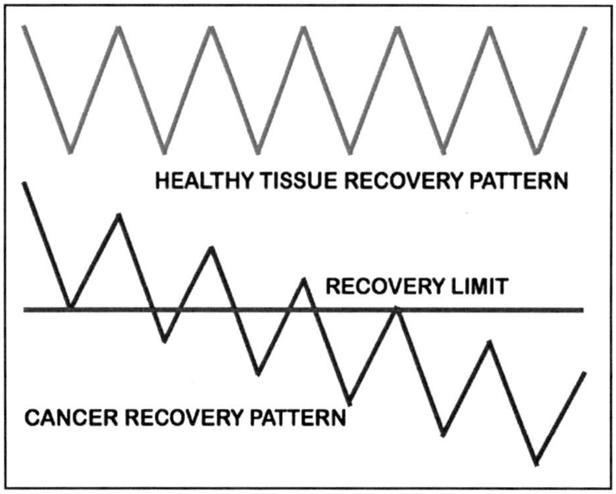

The cancer reaches a point of no recovery.

If healthy tissue recovers after a full dose of proton radiation, then it seems to me that with IMRT, healthy tissue exposed to lower doses should be expected to recover as well. Perhaps extensive exposure to radiation, even at lower levels, produces adverse effects. That would explain why X-rays produce more secondary cancer than proton therapy for some types of cancer, especially for head and throat, and with children—one of the "scary" factors that steered me away from them. Short sighted insurance companies miss the boat by covering only the lower cost IMRT, not taking into consideration the future cost of more secondary prostate cancer and treatment for increased side effects.

A study sponsored by the National Cancer Institute found "a significantly reduced risk" of radiation-induced secondary malignancy with proton therapy. (See: https://www.ncbi.nlm.nih.gov/pmc/articles/PMC4659915/)

Similarly, a study in the United Kingdom reported that 523 (52%) out of every 1,000 new cancer patients are prescribed X-rays as part of their treatment. Out of these, 120 patients (23%) will require re-treatment.

Nancy P. Mendenhall reports in The International Journal of Radiation, Biology, Physics (Vol. 88, Issue 3, pp. 596-602) that IMRT increases the risk of potential recurrence for prostate cancer by *fifteen times*! M. D. Anderson Clinic in Houston calculated for esophageal cancer, X-rays have a whopping 96% additional cancer risk.

The New England Journal of Medicine published a ten-year study of 1,643 men with prostate cancer (September 14, 2016, DOI: 10.1056/NEJMoa1606221.) The study, which divided participants between watchful waiting, surgery, or radiation (X-rays), reached these conclusions.

Of the three treatments, prostatectomy had the greatest negative effect on sexual function and urinary continence, and although there was some recovery, these outcomes remained worse in the prostatectomy group than in the other groups throughout the trial.

"Throughout the trial" means surgery had the worst effects for ten years. That directly contradicts my urologist who waved off surgery as if it were nothing. This ten-year study focused on what were then the three leading treatment modalities, all of which showed some side effects. Had proton therapy been included it almost certainly would have fared much better.

A serious problem arises when doing random blind trials comparing proton therapy to other modalities. You must subject trial participants to lesser and possibly damaging treatments (other than protons) just to prove a point. It violates the basic precept of "first do no harm."

My wife's nephew found himself in just such a dilemma when he was diagnosed with prostate cancer. Offered a chance to be in a blind trial between proton therapy and IMRT, he declined, because he wanted to make sure he would be in the proton group, which they couldn't guarantee since participants get assigned randomly. Such studies find it hard to find enough participants.

The 'rules of evidence' of such random trials are not well-suited to proton therapy in which evidence is mainly related to what proton therapy doesn't do, namely it doesn't damage normal tissue. It's difficult to prove what doesn't happen.

Without the evidence provided by blind trials, critics will continue to call proton therapy experimental and lacking sufficient scientific proof. Eventually, they'll get over it. Some 200,000 patients have been treated with protons worldwide in the past thirty years.

The survey below records how many people report no impact by their cancer treatment. The higher the bar on the graph, the better.

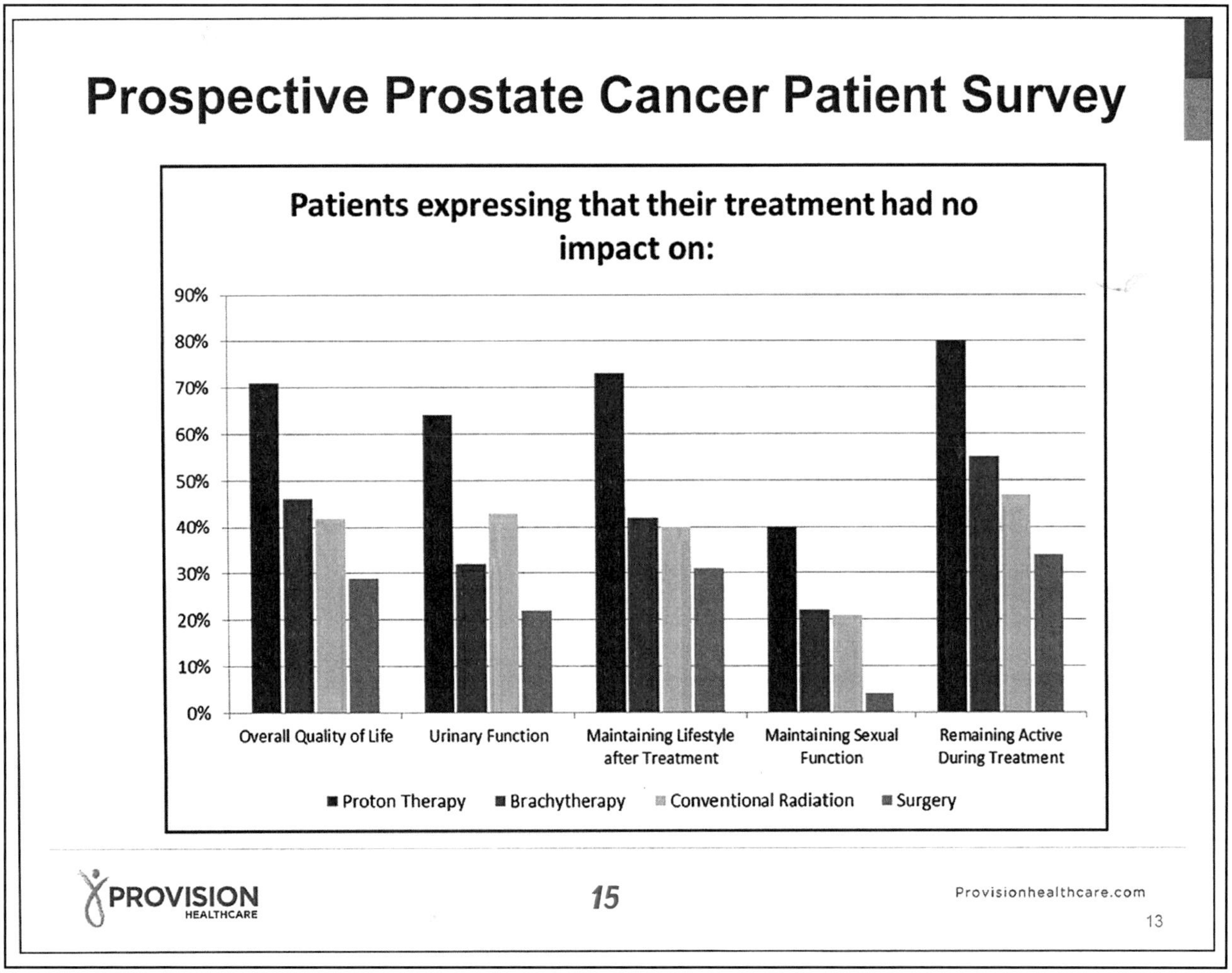

The above chart compares patient-reported impact for protons, brachytherapy (radioactive seeds), conventional radiation, and surgery. This is an attempt to document what didn't happen, which is to say, which modality has the fewest side effects. The higher the bar, the *fewer* the side effects. Note that surgery again comes in last place, X-rays somewhere in the middle, and protons on top.

Note, however, that not even proton therapy patients totally escape impact. The range here, from around 60% to 80%, leaves 40% to 20% of patients with some impact. The most common complication involves urinary function. Swelling can cause restricted flow while temporary internal inflammation can cause burning and increased urgency. There have also been reports of rectal bleeding, but another new technology (shown later) should reduce that probability.

The original technology, called uniform double-scattering, delivers protons in a pattern shaped mechanically to conform to the outline of the target. More recent technology, called pencil beam scanning (PBS), works differently. Instead of hitting the entire target at once, a single beam lays down a series of spots in rows and layers. Picture a glass full of red and white marbles. PBS could hit all of the red (or white) ones while minimally affecting the others, even if they aren't contiguous. That's brilliant. X-rays, eat your heart out. Even double-scattering can't do that.

Now that PBS significantly improves proton therapy delivery, so must statistics that reflect the older technology now be updated. The University of Florida proton facility in Jacksonville, Florida, documented a five-year success rate for prostate cancer of 98% using the older technology. They are now adding another treatment room with PBS. Being far more flexible and precise in its application, it should get results close to 99% recurrence free (at five years).

A new study came out in the midst of my treatment. These excerpts come from the press release on Provision's website.

Provision Healthcare Announces National Survey Results

Men treated for prostate cancer using proton therapy reported significantly better quality of life than other therapy options.

Knoxville, TN (September 27, 2016)

A national survey released today reported that men treated for prostate cancer who received proton therapy reported significantly better quality of life during and after treatment than those treated with brachytherapy, surgery or traditional X-ray therapy. The survey,carried out via phone and online by Bryant Research, profiled 755 men, ages 50-75, who were surveyed at least 12 months after treatment.

Patients who received proton therapy reported the best outcomes for overall quality of life, urinary function, digestive function, sexual function, ability to remain active during treatment, and living life the way they wanted to after treatment. Notably, more than 70% of proton therapy patients reported that treatment did not interfere at all with their overall quality of life.

"These survey results confirm proton therapy's ability to target radiation to the cancer site without damaging surrounding healthy tissue," says Scott Warwick, Vice President of Provision Healthcare. "With proton therapy, patients feel better during treatment and have a better quality of life afterward."

Other notable results included:

- *The proportion of proton therapy patients reporting that their treatment had no impact on their sexual function was almost double that of the next best scoring treatment in this survey.*
- *Ninety-seven (97%) percent of proton therapy patients said they would recommend their treatment to other men with prostate cancer, significantly higher than the other treatment options.*
- *Ninety-seven (97%) percent of proton therapy patients said they would select this same treatment option should they have to make the decision today compared to brachytherapy (68%), conventional radiation therapy (66%), and surgery (58%) patients.*

It doesn't look like surgery, once experienced, holds up very well as a recommended option. While 755 men don't comprise a huge sample, I suspect they are representative. Surveys, after all, take samples designed to reflect the larger population.

Bryant Research conducted this survey under the leadership of Rebecca Bryant, an alumnus of the University of Tennessee and resident of Knoxville. She has received numerous awards for her work, which can be viewed at http://bryant-research.com/html/about.html. I would feel better, however, if Provision had revealed that they sponsored and paid for the survey. I don't think that means the results are questionable, but I think it would be a good move to be transparent about their sponsorship.

I hope this chapter has made its point, especially from a patient's point of view. Now, let's look a little more closely at my personal situation.

CHAPTER 3 MAKING MY DECISION

I heard my wife Linda exclaim from the other room. “Amazing! It’s exactly the same, word for word!”

“What’s the same, Sweetie?” I asked her.

She exclaimed, “Look at this book by Don Denton about getting proton beam therapy. His urologist said the same thing yours did, literally word for word, as if they were following the same script.”

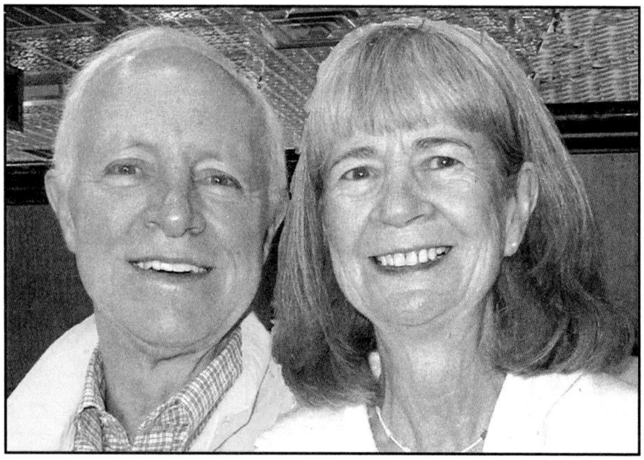

Us.

“That’s pretty much the case,” I told her. “Many other men have heard the same thing.” Shocked, Linda continued quoting from the book she was reading.

“‘I recommend surgery. . . right away . . . the gold standard . . . the best result.’ Denton’s urologist could be quoting yours. I’m shocked.”

“Don’t be,” I replied. “Almost all of them say that. Patients believe it, too. Then they perform the surgery and make lots of money. Virtually all books like this one, written by prostate cancer survivors, broadcast the same message: WAIT. Investigate. Do your research. Be aware of your choices. Don’t let anyone rush you to a decision. Don’t accept uncritically everything they tell you. If your urologist suggests surgery, you’re likely an equally good candidate for proton beam therapy.”

She said, “Urologists have a conflict of interest.”

It’s natural for everyone to promote his or her own specialty: radiation, brachytherapy, surgery, whatever. Rarely do they even mention proton therapy, much less suggest it as a treatment possibility. Dr. Mark Scholz, an oncologist who has treated prostate cancer exclusively for fifteen years, stated in a Maxnews report, “Four out of five operations to remove all or part of the prostate gland are unnecessary.” That amounts to hundreds of thousands of needless surgeries every year and needless suffering. (For the whole article, see: https://www.newsmax.com/health/headline/prostate-surgery-unnecessary-prostate-surgery-prostate-cancer-treatments-for-prostate-cancer/2010/10/18/id/476513/.)

"Urologists have reason to feel threatened," I remarked. "Once the word gets out about protons, some of those surgeons may be working at McDonald's."

"How can anyone know what to do?" Linda asked. "How can they make an informed decision?"

"Many don't," I told her. "They blindly trust their doctor's advice. I'll have to admit, even after I diligently studied all of my options, surgery seemed very attractive. DaVinci robotic equipment looks very impressive. My surgeon's dire prognosis seemed very sincere (and probably was). I eventually made the right choice."

Here's how it happened. On Monday, August 8, 2016, Linda and I met with Dr W. He was young and fit and personable. Not defensive. Admitting the possibility of side effects and lifestyle changes, he told it to me straight.

He said, "It's just a bad situation that you're in. I wish I could make it different. There are no good choices."

I believed him. I didn't yet know that he was wrong. His choices were indeed bad. He continued.

"We'll go wide. We don't want to miss anything. Nerves, margin, seminal vesicles, lymph nodes. And then we'll follow up with radiation."

"Radiation!" I stammered. "Just a few sessions?"

"No," he replied, "a full course."

I couldn't believe it. "Are you kidding me? You want me to do *both* surgery *and* radiation?"

"Exactly." he replied. "You have a very aggressive cancer, so we need to be the same to give you the best survival chance."

I couldn't believe my ears. Dr. W explained. "You stay in the hospital overnight. You go home with a catheter that stays in for a week. You will have a little bag to catch the urine, and a larger one to use at night. Then you will wear pads. After two months, you are likely to be pretty well. Maybe a little leakage here and there. After a year you should be back to normal. Surgery removes one sphincter muscle with the prostate but you have another one. Doing Kegel exercises should strengthen the remaining one. Maybe, if you do something very energetic, you might leak a little from time to time."

"I just worry about wearing diapers for the rest of my life," I admitted. (I like to be frank.)

"No, no," Dr. W assured me. "We wouldn't allow that. We can always go back in and fix things up." (Little did I know how often surgery requires such action.) "We can schedule your surgery for September 14th."

"That's more than five weeks away!" I exclaimed. "What about the cancer growing?"

"We'll be fine anytime within the next two or three months," he said. Months! My head was reeling. I'd been under such pressure to resolve everything. Dr. W said the aggressive cancer required both surgery and radiation, yet there was no hurry. We could wait months? How can that be?

The surgeon's voice stayed in my head: "No good options . . . we'll go wide and take everything." After spending months educating myself, however, I came to two conclusions. First, I wanted proton therapy as the best treatment for my cancer. Second, United Healthcare was unlikely to cover it. I felt I had no other options but to go to Europe and pay for proton therapy out-of-pocket or else submit to surgery followed by radiation.

That same afternoon, August 8, 2016, I got a call from Samantha at Provision CARES Proton Therapy Center in Knoxville, Tennessee. That call changed my life and sent me on the course of adventure and healing described in this book. I made myself a summary of pros and cons to help with my decision.

ROBOTIC SURGERY

Pros

◆ *Costs less than $1,000 out of pocket, covered by insurance, with co-pays*

◆ *Three-hour procedure, one night in hospital, all done*

◆ *I'm in good physical shape, can withstand surgery, would expect a rapid recovery time*

◆ *Recovery time at home in comfortable and familiar surroundings, can get work done (writing, eBay sales)*

◆ *Statistically the best long-term survival rate (this later turns out not to be true)*

◆ *Can examine tissue, determine likely success of procedure*

◆ *Secure in knowledge no prostate cancer remains (also later disproved)*

◆ *Have an extremely well trained, experienced (600 robotic surgeries) and skilled surgeon who does four of these a week*

◆ *Latest DaVinci technology, features 10x magnification, excellent control and accuracy*

◆ *I personally know people who did fine for many years after surgery*

- *Tried and true, not new or unproven*

- *Leaves open a wide range of possible future treatments if necessary*

Cons

- *With radiation follow up, worst combination: two kinds of side effects (surgery and radiation)*

- *Possible secondary cancers*

- *Total loss of erectile function (both nerve bundles removed)*

- *Continence issues, long recovery time, maybe never completely*

- *Over sold, over used (look how many he does!)*

- *Downright frightening*

- *Serious procedure, something could go wrong*

PROTON THERAPY

Pros

- *I determined this to be the best and most advanced technology*

- *Amazed that 80% or more will be covered by Medicare and insurance*

- *Relaxed schedule and more quality time together with Linda*

- *Can write a book about my experience*

- *Not invasive, no recovery time from treatment*

- *Retain sexual function and continence*

- *Minimally lasting side effects*

- *An adventure experiencing treatment of the future*

- *High rate of success*

Cons

- *Still likely to be $15,000 out of pocket*

- *Gone from home, issues with mail, care of house*

- *Hassle and expense of setting up temporary household*

- *Length of treatment*

- *Insecurity that all cancer will be eliminated*

- *Removes surgery as a future salvage treatment if needed*

Since you're holding this book, you know the choice I made. Let's go further back in time and see how I reached the point where I got that life-saving call from Samantha. Her calm assurance and quick response convinced me to go to Knoxville.

CHAPTER 4 DIAGNOSIS

"You've carried watchful waiting far too long," said my urologist. Actually, my delay reflected ignorance. I wasn't being watchful at all. My PSA progressed as follows.

February, 2013:	3.15
January, 2015:	6.46
July, 2015:	6.40
January, 2016:	12.3
May, 2016:	16.0

Three years earlier I should have been more vigilant. The summaries of my blood tests hid the PSA results in obscure places. The right column indicated "high." My cholesterol rated high too, and my blood pressure. I don't recall my family physician saying anything at all about the elevated PSA. Perhaps, like me, he didn't notice it, although for an older man like myself, I should think checking PSA would be standard practice. Somehow, we missed it.

In January, 2016, I changed health plans and doctors. The routine blood test showed a PSA of 12.3. "Holy Toledo, that's high!" Dr. J didn't hide his surprise. Inflammation could have raised my PSA, so he prescribed a round of antibiotics. The May numbers eliminated inflammation as the cause, with the PSA climbing to 16.0. The rapid increase caused alarm.

Dr. J referred me to Dr. H, a urologist. After traveling in June, I reported to him in early July, 2016.

A retired career military doctor now in private practice, Dr. H is tall and forceful, with a firm handshake, a confident manner, and more than a little intimidating. He exhibited shock at my numbers. "Holy Toledo," he said. No, not really. He actually said:

"Biopsy! It's urgent. Can you come in tomorrow morning?"

Shaken by his air of impending disaster, I agreed. However, it couldn't be arranged. Instead, he scheduled me for two weeks later, after his vacation.

When Linda and I arrived for the biopsy, I informed Dr. H that I wanted to wait. "I've been reading," I said, "about a more detailed kind of MRI called a Dynamic Contrast Enhanced (DCE) MRI that can locate the cancer. Then you could do a targeted biopsy."

"I don't need it," he replied instantly. "You have a PSA over sixteen. Certainly you have cancer.

We need a diagnosis before we can begin any kind of treatment."

I tried again. "What about a color Doppler ultrasound to direct your biopsy?"

"I don't need it," he repeated. "That just shows blood flow. I follow a set pattern."

Several books I had read clearly stated that targeted biopsies are superior and more effective. The same for the DCE-MRI. Now Dr. H pooh poohed all of that. He continued:

"I do a randomized biopsy, twelve cores, six on each side, in a grid. The cancer can be microscopic. I wouldn't change my procedure based on a scan."

I shrank into a fog of muddled confusion and dread. What had I done? I thought I understood my options. He didn't care. I'd meddled and messed things up. I felt really stupid as he dismissed my suggestions out of hand.

In my life I have regularly overruled my doctors' prescriptions. I didn't take the Prednisone (a synthetic steroidal hormone) a rheumatologist wanted me to take. Instead, I gave up eating gluten and my arthritis pain went away. A cardiologist recommended I take a statin. No way. I changed my lifestyle and got my cholesterol under control. But cancer was far more serious, life threatening. I thought to myself, "I'm not qualified to make such important decisions; yet I also don't trust everything Dr. H tells me. I think he deliberately exaggerates to make his point. Now I'm really in a fix."

When in the room with Dr. H, I told myself I'd get out of the way this time and be a good patient. I'd follow his advice. But then when I got home and started reading, I couldn't help but question what he said. He seemed to be steeped in an outmoded tradition. I think of his career in the military. Did he just order his patients to do what he said? Would all urologists like to do that? The books I read were written for a purpose, the same as this book, namely, to counter such rampant misinformation.

Much later I read the description that Dr. H typed into my official record.

When the cancer was diagnosed and prior to any treatment, I discussed the significance of the Gleason score edifying this as intermediate-risk disease. In addition, I extensively discussed the types of treatments available to him with regard to his age and overall condition. I further discussed the possible side effects and longevity prospects of each treatment. The patient expressed an understanding of this discussion. He is being (has been) treated with PROTON IN TN 9/16.

Sadly, this is completely fictitious. Nothing of the kind happened. He mentioned only surgery and X-rays, saying I was healthy for my age and should have "no problem" recovering. "Treated with proton." It sounds as if he doesn't even know what it is. I have no idea what 9/16 represents.

"Did you do your preparation for the biopsy?" he asks. "Did you take your antibiotics?"

"No. I didn't expect to do the biopsy today."

He shook his head. I could almost read his mind: "Geez, I've got one of *them*, who does a little research on the internet and thinks he's an expert." But he actually said out loud:

"See my nurse and reschedule as soon as possible. Time is critical. Don't fool around." With that he went to the next exam room to another of his thirty patients that day.

I reported to his heroic insurance administrator, Nancy. She handled referrals, insurance approvals, and the myriad paperwork required these days. I explained about the DCE-MRI. Only one facility in all of San Antonio had that capability, Methodist Hospital, which wasn't in my United Healthcare (AARP Secure Horizons) HMO network. In just five days she got the MRI approved by my insurance (with a twenty percent copay of $400).

Now feeling contrite that I blew my biopsy, I called each day to see if a cancellation had opened up a spot in the schedule. Otherwise, I would have to wait almost a month. On Wednesday I lucked out and snagged a spot the next morning, exactly one week from the aborted biopsy. I was relieved.

Dr. H turned out to be very skilled. I had little discomfort. I could hear the snap of the spring-loaded device and then felt a little nip being removed from my prostate. This time I had taken my antibiotic. For a day or two after the biopsy, I had a little blood in my urine, then I was fine. Horror stories abound regarding biopsies. One friend called it the worst part of his prostate cancer treatment. When we left the office after the biopsy, Linda and I went to Walmart to buy groceries. No big deal.

A few days later, while standing in the vegetable section at H.E.B. grocery store looking at organic avocados, I heard my cellphone ring. I answered with my usual "Robert here."

"This is Dr. H. Your biopsy is positive. Seven of the twelve samples are malignant. Your Gleason score is 4+3=7. That's not good. Call and make an appointment to come in as soon as possible."

"Okay. Thanks." Thanks for what, exactly? While not a surprise, the blunt disclosure still shocked me. Most of the cancer stories I've been reading describe PSA scores of, say, 7.5 as if they were astronomical. They sound piddling next to my 16.0. Linda came over to me and could tell what the call was. I managed to squeak, "Cancer." Then tears by the celery.

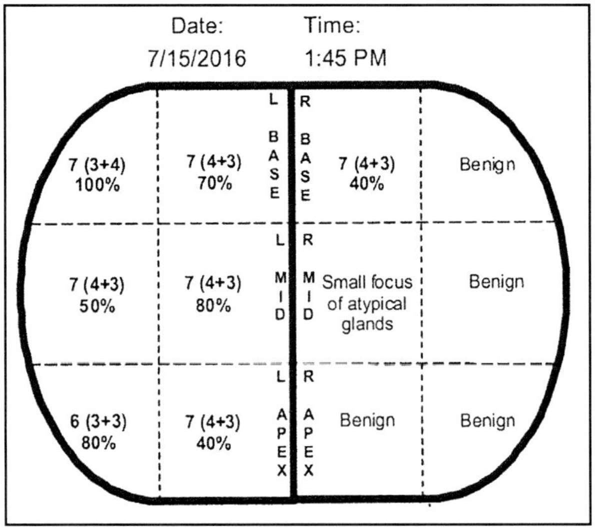

The results of my biopsy.

Some accounts say people become devastated when they receive a cancer diagnosis, especially with no symptoms or warning. I'm very happy with my life but was disturbed that I'd waited so long. That complicated things. A full report of the biopsy comes in the mail, along with a diagram locating the positive cores, predominantly on the left side. It gave a percentage for each core.

It just made no sense at all. I don't know of any history of prostate cancer in my family. I'm healthy and robust, with a healthy lifestyle. What did I do to deserve this? How did it happen?

A few days later, on my seventy-second birthday (July 21, 2016), I had the DCE-MRI. In my documentation the medical staff noticed the coincidence. "Happy birthday." "Thanks." Then my attempt at humor. "Birthdays are good for longevity. People with the most birthdays live the longest." They didn't laugh. Oh, well. They were busy working. The results of the MRI said the following:

1. Small focus of double match (decreased T2 signal and diffusion restriction) in the medial left peripheral zones in mid gland, suggestive of primary prostate malignancy. Dynamic contrast enhancement in this location is not overly suspicious, however.

2. No evidence of extracapsular extension. No suspicious pelvic lymphadenopathy.

The DCE-MRI showed that the cancer had *not* spread beyond the prostate. Hallelujah! That opened up many more viable treatment options. Much relieved, I returned to my studies with new intensity and urgency. I needed to make a decision before the cancer spread.

A week after the DCE-MRI, I had a full-body bone scan. When prostate cancer spreads, it tends to go to the bones. In such case, it remains prostate cancer, just located elsewhere. It isn't bone cancer. My friend Jeff was diagnosed with advanced metastatic prostate cancer. He told me his bone scan "lit up like a Christmas tree." After my scan, the technician couldn't give results, but indicated I would be pleased. Then he asked a question.

"What's going on in your left jaw?"

"I have no idea."

"Well, something's not right there."

So the next day I went to my dentist and learned I had a serious infection in my lower left jaw, which led to having a root canal. I never would have known until things had gotten much more out of hand. It gave me confidence in the integrity of the bone scan.

A few days later I received this report.

FINDINGS
3 hour delayed anterior and posterior whole body images were performed. Nominal distribution of radiotracer. Focus of moderately intense activity in the left mandible. Faint degenerative activity noted in both shoulders, both knees, and both feet. Symmetrical renal activity is noted.

IMPRESSION
1. Focus of abnormal activity in the left mandible likely related to dental disease or recent procedure. Clinical correlation requested.
2. No evidence of skeletal metastatic disease.

Let's repeat: I had no skeletal metastatic disease, even after reaching serious PSA numbers. Once the cancer escapes the prostate, the five-year survival rate sinks to around thirty percent. But not for me. Unbelievable. Miraculous.

In my reading I found *An ABC of Prostate Cancer in 2015: My Journey Over 4 Continents to Find the Best Cure*, by Alan G. Lawrenson. (There is now a more recent update available.) A medical researcher in Australia, he describes the various treatment options with the kind of details for which I hungered. In the end, he chooses proton therapy. As it isn't covered by his insurance company, he goes to Seoul, South Korea, where he pays half as much.

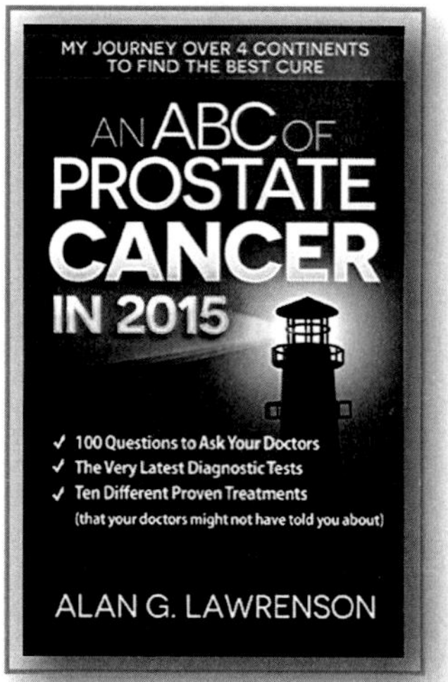

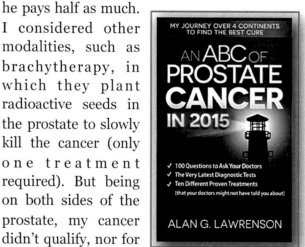

I considered other modalities, such as brachytherapy, in which they plant radioactive seeds in the prostate to slowly kill the cancer (only one treatment required). But being on both sides of the prostate, my cancer didn't qualify, nor for other treatments like focal laser ablation that treats only part of the prostate. I needed the whole gland addressed. So, like Alan, my analysis settled on proton therapy.

I contemplated going to Korea. Then I discovered Prague, where proton therapy takes just twenty-one rather than thirty-nine sessions. Two years ago it cost about $33,000, plus travel, lodging and expenses, likely $40,000 all told. Sounded romantic. I investigated lodging but nothing looked right. Many people would welcome six weeks in Prague. Being older, however, I found everything seemed too difficult, with language barriers, shopping for food, cooking, transportation, and so forth.

Brooke Palmer in Prague (an American from Alabama) spent a lot of time answering my many email questions. The proton center has a British office and website to channel people there from England (covered by insurance). Brooke was very helpful and encouraging. I was recently in touch with the Prague center again when they responded to my request for graphics by sending some of the illustrations you will find in this book. I have a very good feeling about them.

Back to my story. Next, I called several proton centers in the United States, asking what my out-of-pocket cost would be. The University of Florida in Jacksonville quoted $160,000; but for all cash, they would discount it to $134,000. Several other places, including M. D. Anderson, wouldn't give me a price over the telephone without having a consultation first, in person. This was not possible.

On Friday, August 5, 2016 I sent out emails to twelve proton therapy centers, mostly in the United States, a few in Europe. I received negative answers from France and Sweden. A new center in Irving (Dallas), Texas, sent me a fancy packet by overnight Express Mail, received on Saturday. Very cool. They understood how urgently I wanted to receive information.

On the following Monday, Linda and I met with the prospective surgeon, Dr. W, followed that afternoon by Samantha's call from Provision in Knoxville.

"Here's the problem," I told her. "My insurance won't pay for it. How much will it cost out of pocket?"

"Are you on Medicare?"

"Well, yes. I have an Advantage HMO plan but it explicitly doesn't cover proton therapy. I'm trying to find out how much a treatment will cost me."

I know how advantage plans work. The insurance company takes over all responsibility for my covered health costs from Medicare for which they receive a set fee (something like $11,000 year, maybe more). To make a profit, they must deliver care for less than that. So they have a conflict of interest. They want to spend as little on me as possible.

A few years ago, I went into my doctor with a temperature and congestion. He suggested that I might have the flu. The next day I flew to

Puerto Vallarta, Mexico, for my annual timeshare visit. I figured that would be a good place to recover. However, when I went to see the hotel doctor, he called an ambulance and rushed me to the hospital with a very serious case of double pneumonia. My HMO had performed no tests of any kind, presumably to save money. While hospitalized for three days in Mexico I received far better treatment than anything I would expect at home, at a fraction of the cost. Including scans, doctor's fees, room, meals, and everything else, the bill was $8,000. Only after a battle did my insurance eventually reimburse me.

Proton therapy costs many times what United Healthcare receives for my care; so they won't cover it unless absolutely forced to do so.

To my question about cost, Samantha replied:

Robert,

Just to give you an idea, the cash rates for the protocol using 39 treatments would be around $93,600. We also offer a hypo-fractionation protocol which is only 20 treatments which would be around $48,000. We are also offering the 20 treatment protocol in a clinical trial. We have actually seen several commercial insurance carriers more willing to pay for the hypofractionation protocol since the actual cost is very comparable to IMRT. My finance team can also work out payment plans and other options if your insurance truly doesn't cover treatment for proton therapy.

What insurance do you have? I'd be happy to have my finance team look into your coverage for you as well. Do you know if your plan is self-funded? My finance team can look at your policy to see if they think there is any way to get proton therapy covered for you based on the language in your policy. My finance team are huge advocates for our patients, and I know they have been able to get around 30% of cases, on average, approved when the patient's insurance policy states that proton therapy is "not medically necessary." I think it would at least be worth taking a look at to see if they think it may be possible for us to get treatment approved for you.

As far as outcomes with proton therapy, studies have shown that patients in the intermediate risk level you described as having a 96% to 99% cure rate with proton therapy, which is even higher than the national average cure rate. Our staff here in Knoxville have around 300 years of experience in proton therapy, which is far more than any other proton center in the US. We have an outstanding team and center in Knoxville, and I'd love to help see if this could be a viable option for you. Please feel free to email me or call me with any questions or concerns.

She presented many possible options, including fewer treatments at a lower cost. Three hundred years of experience! Impressive. She put me in touch with Steve in the finance department who assured me that if I would participate in a registry to track the results of my proton therapy, Medicare would cover 80% of my cost for proton therapy. It sounded too good to be true. I continued to question whether I understood what they were saying.

"I don't understand, Steve. Medicare? Directly? I'm in an HMO network. Medicare would pay directly, outside of United Healthcare?"

"Yes. If you're willing to be included in our registry trial for patients treated with proton beam therapy, Medicare will pay 80% of your cost."

Spectacular. On the morning of August 10, I received a call from Dr. Marcio Fagundes, then medical director of Provision, to answer any questions I might have. We discussed all of my numbers, which indicated that I qualify for proton beam therapy. Meanwhile, Rhonda Turner, manager of patient financial services, responded to my continued amazement at the possibility that I won't have to pay for treatment myself. She wrote:

> *Thank you so very much for speaking with me this morning. I hope that I have answered your questions and put your concerns to rest. You will see I have attached a copy of our local Medicare coverage policy and I have highlighted the areas that pertain to your case. Please do not hesitate to reach out to me if I can assist you in any other way. Have a blessed rest of the week!*

So important is this information for all men on Medicare that I have dedicated an entire chapter to it (see page 88).

On August 10, two days after first contact, I filled out the patient admission forms. I also sent by overnight express the CDs for my bone scan and DCE-MRI. Dr. Fagundes wanted me to take hormones for three or four months, waiting four to six weeks before starting treatment. I really struggled with that. It would delay my treatment until October and November. Bummer.

Androgens, mainly testosterone, feed prostate cancer. Hormone therapy deprives or suppresses these androgens, making the tumor(s) shrink and become much less active, therefore, easier to treat. Most testosterone is made in the testicles. Surgically removing them solves the problem. However, castration would be irreversible with permanent side effects. Hormones achieve chemical castration, reaching the same goal, but one can stop taking them and end the side effects. Hormones don't kill cancer; they just delay its growth. Depending on how old you are, that may be enough. As they say, many more men die *with* prostate cancer than *of* it.

Lupron was the hormone of choice. The potential side effects include fast or irregular heart beat (I already have that), sudden decrease in blood pressure and collapse, blurred vision, joint pain, unusual bleeding or bruising, cough, diarrhea, loss of appetite, runny nose, shivering, insomnia, erectile disfunction and more. Whew!

I looked up the circumstances that call for hormones. They include the following:

a. If the cancer has spread too far to be cured by surgery or radiation, or if you can't have these treatments for some other reason.

b. If the cancer remains or comes back after treatment with surgery or radiation therapy.

c. Along with radiation therapy as initial treatment if you are at higher risk of the cancer coming back after treatment (based on a high Gleason score, high PSA level, and/or growth of the cancer outside the prostate).

d. Before radiation to try to shrink the cancer to make treatment more effective.

These applied to me only peripherally. A Gleason of 4+3=7 wasn't outrageously high, although a PSA of 16.0 certainly was. The fourth reason (d) most closely reflected the doctor's intent. Samantha tried to calm my unrest, writing:

> *I have actually had Lupron injections before, and I did the monthly injections, and all the information online was very scary and intimidating, but personally, the only changes I noticed were having hot flashes, especially worse if I had a glass of wine. With that being said, you and I are completely different people, so I don't know if you'll have an experience like I had or see and experience other things. Most of the gentlemen I have spoken with here that had to go through hormone therapy only spoke to having occasional hot flashes and a few noticed slight irritability.*

Over several days we had a flurry of telephone calls and emails. I apologized for being so resistant. Samantha was understanding.

> *I think getting all your questions answered and objectively looking at everything is very important to decision making for treatment and knowing that you're making the right decision for treatment, and I want to help make sure that you have the confidence you need in knowing that the treatment you're doing is truly the best thing for you.*

I talked later in the day with Dr. Fagundes and he approved me as a good prospect for proton therapy, *without* the need for hormones. He said in the long run, the difference between using hormones or not affects the survival rate by a couple of percentage points from, say, 95% to 93%. I affirmed that I accepted the slight additional risk. Soon, we were on our way.

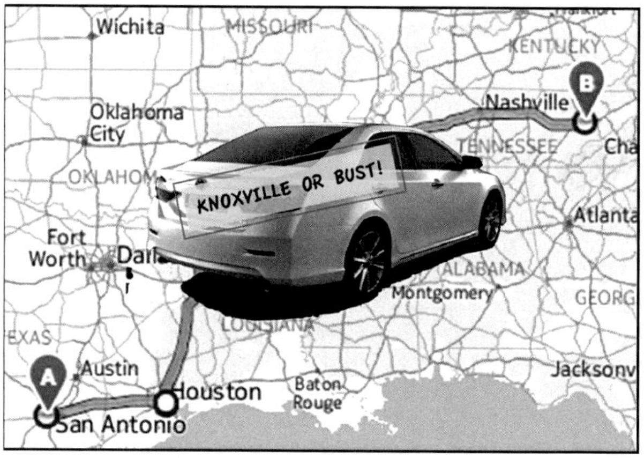

We arrived in Knoxville on August 31, 2016.

CHAPTER 5 GETTING STARTED

The hospitality team at Provision helped us find a lovely two-bedroom furnished cottage on Deane Hill Drive, just three miles from Provision and only blocks from Kingston Pike, a long commercial thoroughfare filled with businesses, restaurants, and everything we could need. The owner of the house himself had previously survived prostate surgery.

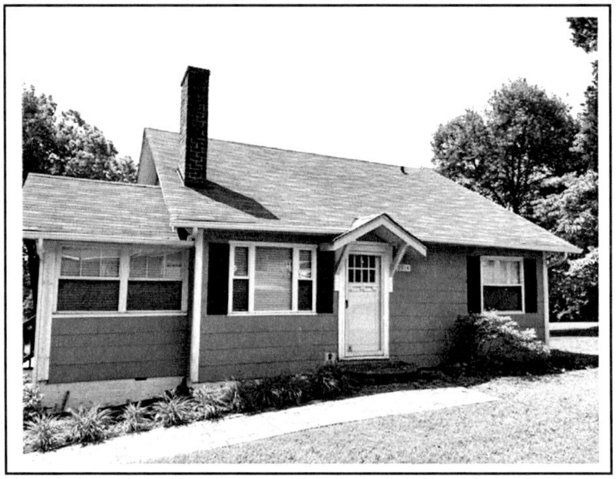

Everything in our abode was new: shingles on the roof, fresh paint inside and out, floors refinished. Appliances, towels, furniture, cooking utensils, hardy no-stick pots and pans, rugs, bed linen; everything was brand shiny new. The back deck looked out at a two-acre field, while the front of the house faced a busy street.

The house had an alarm system and room to turn around in the driveway to avoid backing into the street. All of this at a reasonable cost. We couldn't have asked for more.

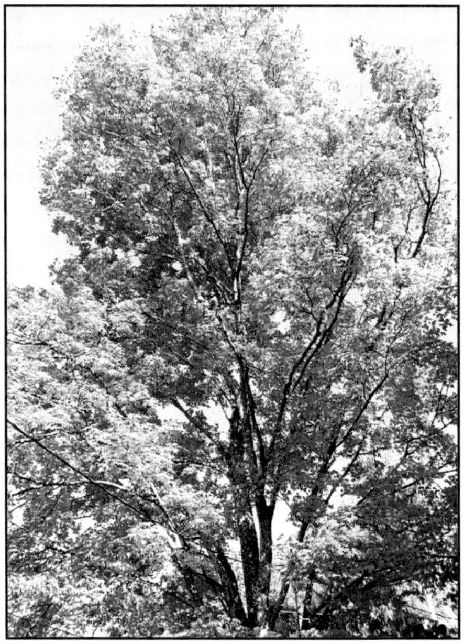

The tree at the end of the driveway.

We were less than a mile from Whole Foods, Trader Joe's, and a restaurant we like called Bonefish. We got free library cards for the Bearden branch, just blocks away, checking out numerous books. Traversing the three miles to Provision took about ten minutes to drive each morning, without needing to use a busy highway. It took a few minutes longer if the lights were red.

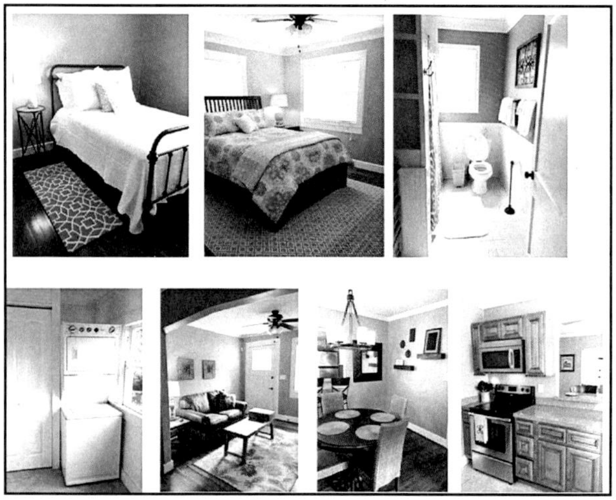

Interior of Deane Hill Cottage.

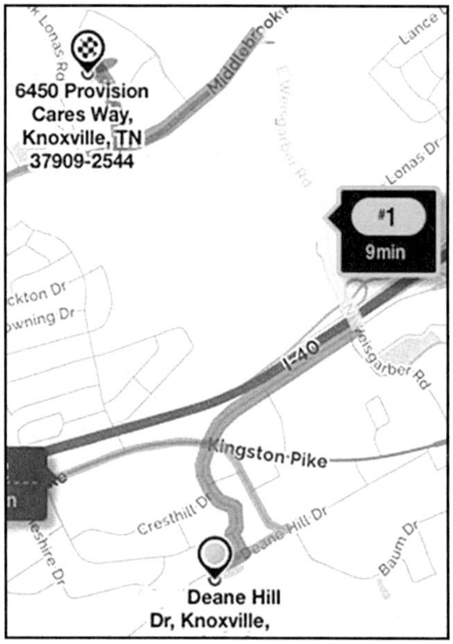

The route to Provision..

On September 1, 2016, we arrived early to check the layout of the campus, including a winding trail along a tumbling water course. Ten minutes before my 11:00 o'clock appointment, I posed for a photo at the front door. Then we went in.

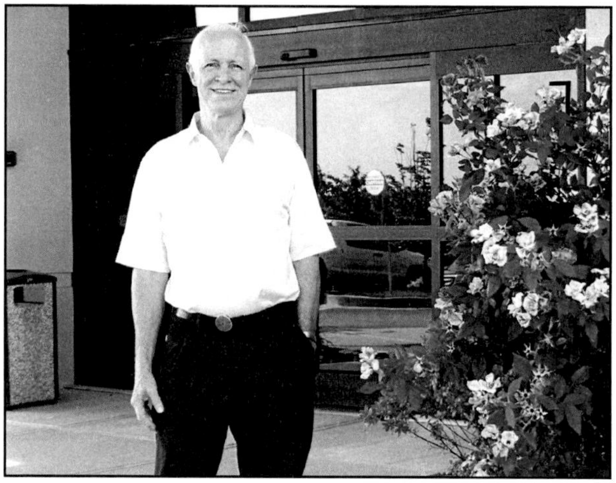

First arriving at Provision, smiling but apprehensive.

Sharon Hall greeted us from the front desk. In the subsequent two months, she would be our interface with the staff and all the resources I required to write this book. She took a photo for my badge after which I met with several people to do required paperwork for my treatment. Everything had been prearranged and went smoothly. I felt confident in relaxing and trusting the process.

I signed many documents: Medicare coverage, joining the cancer registry for proton therapy, insurance coverage (details about my policy with United Healthcare), a Financial Policy form and a Patient Payment Plan. I signed an acknowledgement for having received notice of their privacy practices, a HIPAA authorization and a scheduling document. I signed a Patient Responsibility Summary, an Advanced Beneficiary Notice of Non-coverage for the SpaceOAR (more on that later), and yet another HIPAA authorization.

A nurse went over my medical history and informed me of my schedule for the two days of preparation. She registered my blood pressure as 159/93. I guess I was a little nervous.

Ever diligent, I had started preparing a week earlier. Besides a blow-by-blow account of what to expect in the preparation stage, I previously received a sheet about dietary restrictions to avoid intestinal gas. It forbade some of my favorite and healthiest foods. (More on this later.) The instructions also restricted any form of blood thinners, aspirin or NSAIDs.

After this meeting ended, the time arrived to perform my Fleet enema, supposedly two hours prior to the doctor's procedures. However, by then it was 1:00 p.m. and the appointment was at 2:00 o'clock. The nurse assured me that would be acceptable. She gave me some pills to take, including Valium to relax me, Hydrocodone/Tylenol for pain relief, and an antibiotic. She also applied EMLA numbing cream to the perineum area. It became eminently clear to me that treatment in this part of the body quickly divests you of any sense of privacy or embarrassment.

Upon learning that I would need an enema, I had originally pictured a bag of fluid hanging high in the air with a tube running from it and a clamp to turn the flow on and off. That had been my previous experience. I once tried a wheatgrass enema, with rather hilarious (and very green) results.

Fleet makes an enema simpler, easier, and civilized. It comes in a 4.5 ounce plastic bottle with a long tip. The box gives numerous warnings and contraindications. Don't do more than one within twenty-four hours. Get a doctor's input if you are over fifty-five years old. Beware if you are on a sodium-restricted diet, as the bottle contains sodium phosphate, a saline solution. It apparently works by increasing fluid in the small intestine, causing a bowel movement within one to five minutes. I had in my bag two Fleet enema bottles that I had purchased at CVS pharmacy.

I went to a small examination room located next to the men's room. After reading the instructions twice, I assumed a position on my knees with my head by the floor and my rear end in the air. I removed the protective shield and inserted the narrow "pre-lubricated comfortip" (right!) in the designated place. Working behind me, I couldn't see what I was doing. I began squeezing the bottle. When full, it felt solid, but it was actually very flimsy so it could collapse when the contents went out through the one-way valve.

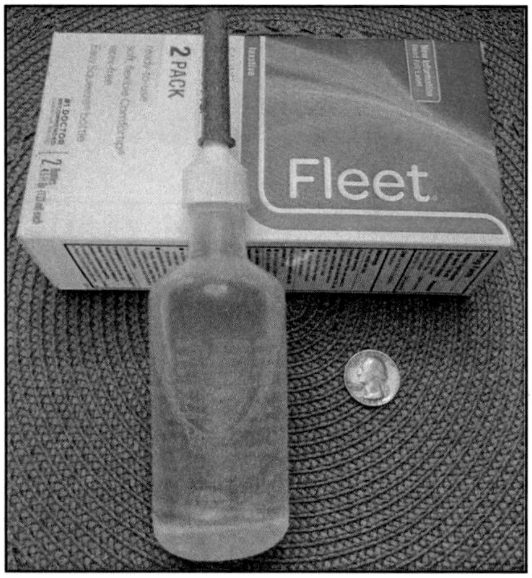

Fleet enema, two bottles per package.

Thinking I was finished, I removed the bottle and looked at it, shocked to see it remained half full. So I reassumed the position and reinserted the bottle to squeeze out more of the contents.

I casually dressed and removed myself to the men's room, not very impressed by what I produced. I fastened my pants and washed my hands, ready to leave when a major cramp hit me. Oh, I wasn't finished. Finally successful, I went back to the lobby until appointment time. No lunch.

The lobby overflows with comfortable lounge chairs arranged in small groups to enhance interaction with other patients, rather like a living room. We became friends with people whom we saw every day. Conversation often centered around our various treatments or other medical issues.

I remember visiting a cancer clinic in Bad Mergantheim, Germany, that had signs throughout the facility instructing "do not talk to others about your illness or condition, it doesn't help you or them." They want patients to keep a positive outlook and to expect the best, not share horror stories. Still, I asked others about their experiences with their treatment and their urologist. People seemed willing and interested in sharing.

Let's get right to our anatomy lesson. A year ago I couldn't have even described the prostate.

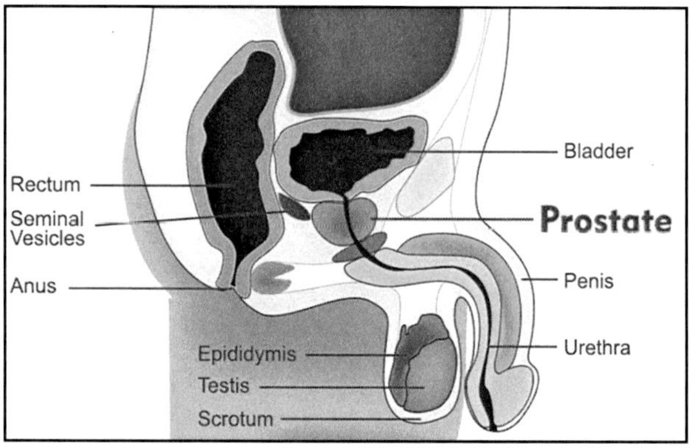

The prostate rests below the bladder and in front of the rectum. It surrounds part of the urethra, the tube that carries urine from the bladder. I think the rectum is more immediately adjacent to the prostate than shown here. Otherwise, there would be no reason to protect it (see SpaceOAR on page 36).

In 2011 Laurence Roy Stains won an award from the American Society of Magazine Editors for a clever article about his prostate experience in *Men's Health Magazine*. Here's an excerpt.

Your prostate gland labors in obscurity. The size of a golf ball, it's tucked away under your bladder, biding its time until you and your reproductive system decide to emit the sacred seed. Then the semen assembly line kicks in: The sperm swim up from your testicles to the seminal vesicles, and there they are mixed in a happy bath of fructose, vitamin C, and prostaglandins. This brew then proceeds to your prostate, which tops it off with enzymes, citric acid, and zinc before your man milk is propelled out of your body and into hers with rather pleasant smooth-muscle contractions. This long bomb triumphantly delivers your DNA into the end zone. (For the entire article, see: https://www.menshealth.com/health/a19540939/coping-with-prostate-cancer/)

Stains didn't reveal why there need to be hundreds of thousands of sperm in each ejaculation to reach one egg. The reason is . . . they don't like to ask for directions!

After a short wait, I donned a backless gown and went to a small room where two nurses hooked me up to machines that monitor my blood pressure and pulse. They arranged me on a table on my back with my legs high in the air, held by two devices designed for that purpose. For a moment I thought I had made a wrong turn and ended up in a gynecologist's office.

They placed a rolled up towel under my scrotum and penis to lift everything up and out of the way, making the perineum accessible. A small towel offered a modicum of privacy.

Dr. Fagundes cames into the room and said hello. I noticed the nurses kept up a conversation with me, perhaps to distract me from what was happening. Dr. Fagundes gave me a shot through the perineum to numb the prostate. He then proceeded to place three small gold chains called fiducials into my prostate. (I'm glad they are permanent, as trying to remove them would be very damaging.) A small ultrasound probe in my rectum gave a clearer image of my prostate. The three points are non-collinear, which means none will visually overlap when viewed from any direction.

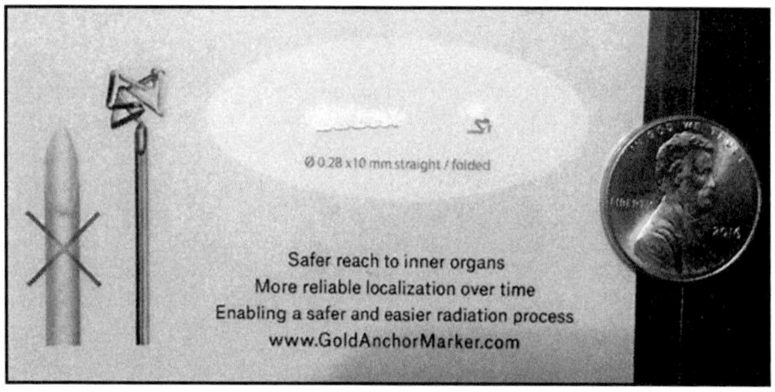

This card contains the kind of fiducial markers I received, two straight and one bent (folded). The penny gives a sense of scale. Later I saw how the fiducials looked in my X-rays (see page 43).

Dr. Fagundes announced each placement. "Here goes the first one." From Brazil, he first did proton therapy at Harvard Medical School, later coming to Provision from ProCure Proton Therapy Center in Oklahoma. He announced the second and the third fiducials in the same way, taking perhaps fifteen minutes total. He inserted the fiducial markers into the prostate through the perineum, between the scrotum and the anus. He assured me that he used thin needles, the size of acupuncture needles, not large ones, as when I had my biopsy. I felt no pain.

Meanwhile, the nurse reported my blood pressure as 192/105, the highest I've ever recorded. They told me one man's blood pressure soared well above 200 and wouldn't come down, sending him to the hospital.

Dr. Fagundes then performed a second procedure to inject a gel called SpaceOAR Hydrogel (space between **O**rgan **A**t **R**isk). I read about this in a book by Alan G. Lawrenson from Australia, describing his proton therapy treatment in South Korea. At that time, SpaceOAR wasn't yet used in the United States.

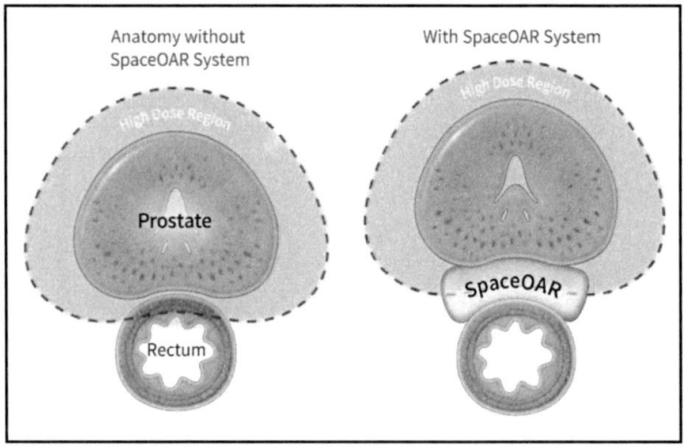

The diagram shows how the gel pushes the rectum away from the prostate and out of reach of the radiation. It remains in place for three months, after which it slowly exits the body in the patients' urine—leaving nothing behind. Illustration used with permission. For more information see the SpaceOAR website at https://www.spaceoar.com/

It took about five minutes to inject the gel, which I found unpleasant, but the discomfort went away quickly. During the next two months, I received CT scans on several occasions to check the location of the gel and fiducial markers. They remained where they were meant to be.

Two years ago insurance didn't cover SpaceOAR; so it cost me three thousand dollars out-of-pocket, a very pricey blob of gel. As of January, 2018, there is a new CPT billing code for SpaceOAR (#55874) used to bill Medicare. That's good news. Maybe it's covered now.

When the FDA approved SpaceOAR in 2015, Provision began using it one week later. In October of 2015, Dr. Fagundes addressed the American Society for Radiation Oncology (ASTRO) at their convention in San Antonio about the benefits of SpaceOAR.

If not using the gel, they insert a balloon into the rectum and fill it with saline water. It helps stabilize the prostate from the rectum side and consistently produces the same position for every treatment. (The bladder content also remains consistent for the same reason.) After thirty-nine balloons, the rectum can get a little sore. Some men don't choose to use the hydrogel because of cost. I later learned that forty percent of Provision's prostate cancer patients still use the balloon. Ouch.

Fifteen years ago, Robert Marckini (whose book is still a major seller) established a support organization called the Brotherhood of the Balloon (BOB). Its website is now owned by Loma Linda University, where he was treated (the first facility to offer proton beam therapy). Now, that name will become an anachronism, like the Brotherhood of the Buggy Whip (BOBW). Perhaps I will start the **B**rotherhood **o**f the **G**el (BOG) or perhaps **B**rotherhood **o**f **S**pace**OAR** **(**BOSOAR**)**. Actually, they could keep their acronym by changing their name to **B**rotherhood **o**f the **B**eam.

The prostate is located such that proton beams skim just under the bladder and within the SpaceOar gel. The balloon, on the other hand, while stabilizing the prostate also pushes the rectum right up against it, virtually assuring that it will receive some of the radiation resulting in possible bowel issues (colitis, etc.). With SpaceOAR, the likelihood of adverse effects is much smaller.

My procedures complete, I regained my dignity and rejoined Linda in the lobby. Together we reviewed the post-fiducial instructions. Avoid heavy exercise for forty-eight hours. I might notice a little blood in my urine or stool, as after my biopsy. (I did, but only for one day.) To protect the SpaceOAR gel, avoid activities that put pressure on the perineum, such as bicycling or riding a horse. No problem. Avoid medical procedures involving the rectal cavity. I had no such plans. Call the doctor if experiencing a temperature over 101 degrees or severe pain. Will do. Thus ended our first day at Provision.

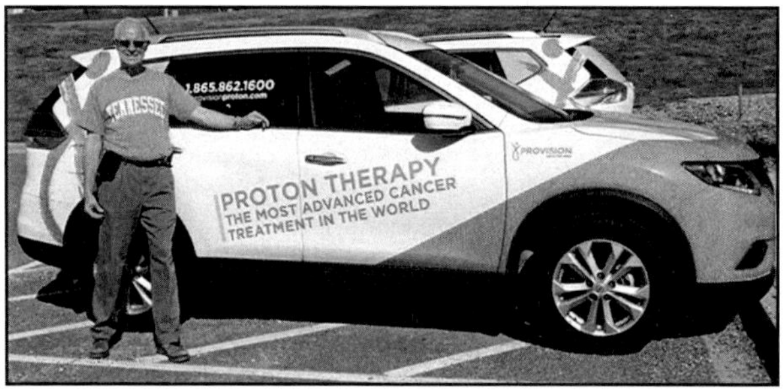

We soon learned that Knoxville goes nuts over the University of Tennessee football team. I duly bought a Tennessee T-shirt. In the parking lot we noticed that the Provision cars are orange and white, Tennessee colors. This didn't happen by accident. The founder of Provision went to the university here for undergraduate, master's and doctoral degrees. Saturday afternoons Knoxville looks like a ghost town while everyone watches or attends the game.

I returned to Provision the next day for two scans. One hour before the Computed Tomography (CT) scan, I emptied my bladder and drank a sixteen ounce bottle of water. At the appointed time, I again donned a backless gown and was taken to the scan room where I lay down on the table with my legs in a kind of tray that they used to make a mold of my legs and feet.

During each of my thirty-nine treatments, this cradle immobilized my lower body and kept it in the same exact position. I saw a video of someone at Loma Linda whose cradle stretched from the neck down and was called a pod. Once my legs fit snugly in my lower body cradle, the prostate couldn't really be out of place.

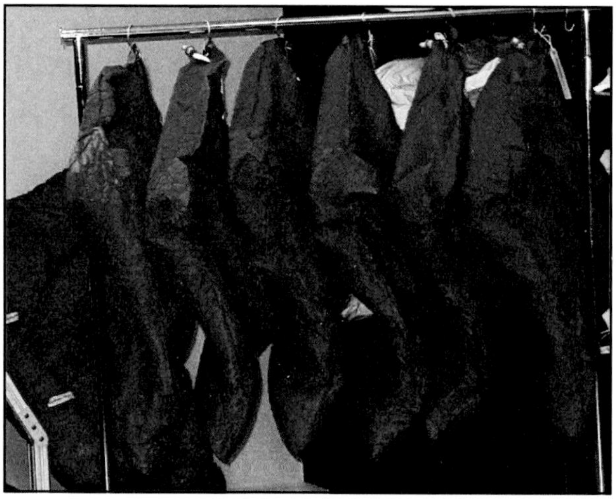

Leg cradles for each patient (inside their protective bags). They recycle the material for making future cradles.

Next they put a tiny dot on each upper thigh, a permanent tattoo used to properly align the proton equipment. Finally I had a tattoo! (You will see a photo of it later.) I can barely find it among the other little dots and freckles. I guess I should go and get something pierced now, as well.

Once I was immobilized and marked in what will be my standard position, a scan records the exact location of my fiducial markers. This whole process, called the simulation, wasn't the actual treatment, just the set up. The techs paused while they sent the image of the scan to Dr. Fagundes for his approval, which they received in five minutes. One scan down, one more to go.

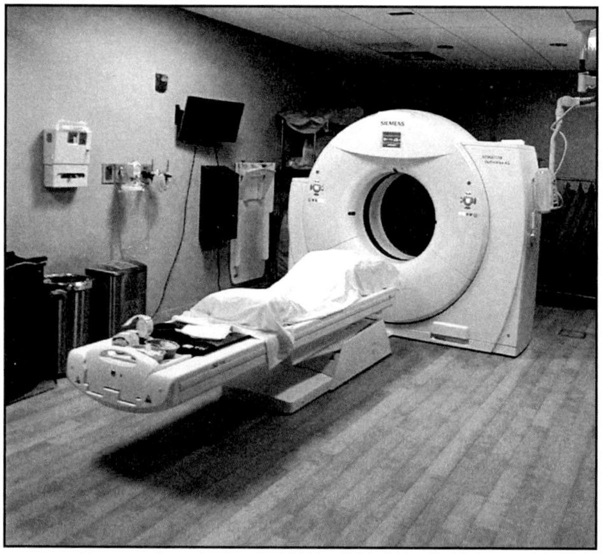

CT scan room

The MRI took place in a different building at an imaging center across the street, where Provision first began. The MRI involved a series of five scans, varying from thirty seconds to ten or so minutes. I lay on the table, which moved forward and backward, wearing headphones to protect my ears from the noise. I chose New Age music.

The MRI and CT scans were fused together to give the best view of the prostate. It takes the dosimetrists a week, sometimes more, to calculate the exact program for the protons. I have dedicated a whole chapter to this subject (page 69).

We timed our arrival in Knoxville to avoid driving over the Labor Day weekend. My two days of preparation procedures took place on Thursday and Friday with the following Monday being a holiday.

Knowing our situation as out-of-towners, they worked up my program in two days. My first treatment took place on Thursday, September 8, 2016, exactly one month after that fateful day of August 8 on which I both talked to the surgeon and received the first call from Samantha.

As I update the first edition of this book, it is rather striking to relive my experience almost two years ago. I never could have predicted my subsequent involvement with proton therapy.

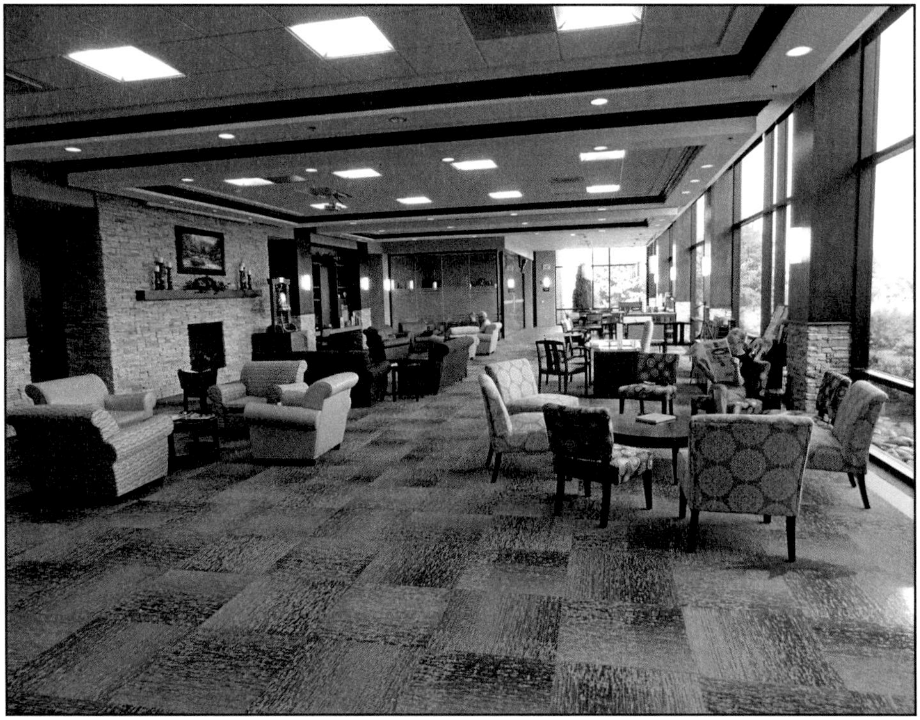

Lobby waiting room.

CHAPTER 6 A TREATMENT DAY

Most mornings I arose at 6:00 a.m., tiptoeing out of the room to avoid waking Linda (usually without success). I attempted to start the day with some quiet contemplation, but my mind was so involved in the treatment process and in writing this book that it was hard to tame.

The morning was organized around my treatment time of 10:20 a.m.. Three hours earlier I could have a light meal, which meant breakfast from 7:00 to 7:15. I then had an hour to look at email or work on my writing, leaving home at 8:15 a.m. Despite rush hour traffic, it typically took only ten minutes or so to get to the Provision campus.

It's located in a commercial development called Dowell Springs. I was once involved in real estate development, so I appreciated the quality evident there, with plenty of open space, more than sufficient parking, water features, walking trails, and sidewalks, plus Provision has its own waterfall and pond.

We parked beside the Provision Wellness Center in one of the tree-shaded parking places, a habit aquired from living in Texas.

From my journal:

I love walking with Linda in Dowell Springs in the mornings, before I work out at the fitness center, shower, and then go for my treatment. There are a variety of routes to walk. A winding trail follows the water feature, cutting back and forth on little bridges. The sidewalk goes up one street, across the top of the hill by the huge F.B.I. building, and then down the other street. That's a bit hard, so Linda doesn't wear her weighted vest when we walk the hill. Alternatively, there's a trail in the woods near some old historical buildings. No one uses that trail, which dead ends. I need to carry a stick to knock down cobwebs across the path. Most often we walk the parking lots. There's a sprawling office condo building surrounded on all sides by parking lot. Three times around takes twenty-five minutes, our usual walking time.

The walk is just our warm up. We then go inside the Wellness Center to the fitness rooms where I use weights and machines while Linda does machines, mat exercises, or classes. In the midst of my workout, at 9:15 a.m., an hour before treatment, I empty my bladder and drink sixteen ounces of water within five minutes. Usually, I just gulp it down in about twenty seconds.

I then continue to work out, followed by a leisurely shower (there's rarely anyone else in the locker room). I use the handicapped shower because it's roomier. I get dressed and walk over to Provision across the street for my treatment, feeling clean, energized and ready for the world. Linda stays at the Wellness Center for a yoga class or to write in her journal.

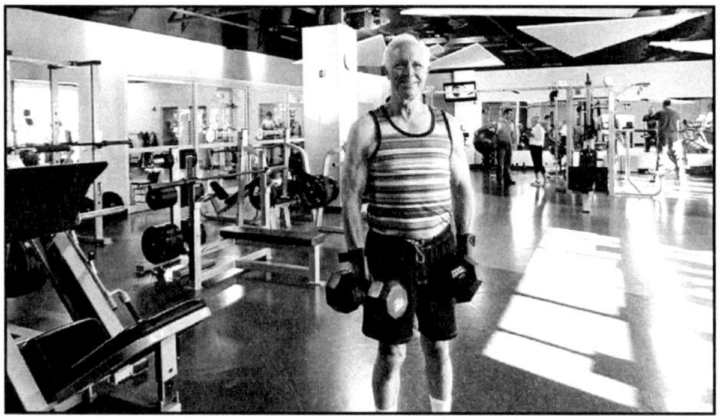

At the Wellness Center: One of two large rooms filled with equipment including treadmills, machines, and free weights as well as various devices like medicine balls and stretchy bands.

Upon entering Provision, I went to the front desk, said hello to Sharon and placed the back of my name badge under the scanner until it beeped, recording my personal barcode. Now the system knew that I'd arrived. On the days that Linda came to Provision with me, we usually walked to the end of the lobby and sat at one of the tables where we wrote in our journals. If Linda stayed at the Wellness Center, then I sat in one of the grouped lounge chairs and talked to people.

There were also women there, undergoing treatment for breast or other cancers. There were almost as many women as men. That Linda accompanied me every day was a wonderful gesture of support.

At 10:15 a technician came out to the lobby to get me, taking me to changing room Autumn One. I removed my clothes from the waist down and donned a gown. Then I put on the special socks that I wore for all my treatments. I became known as the guy with the hot pepper socks.

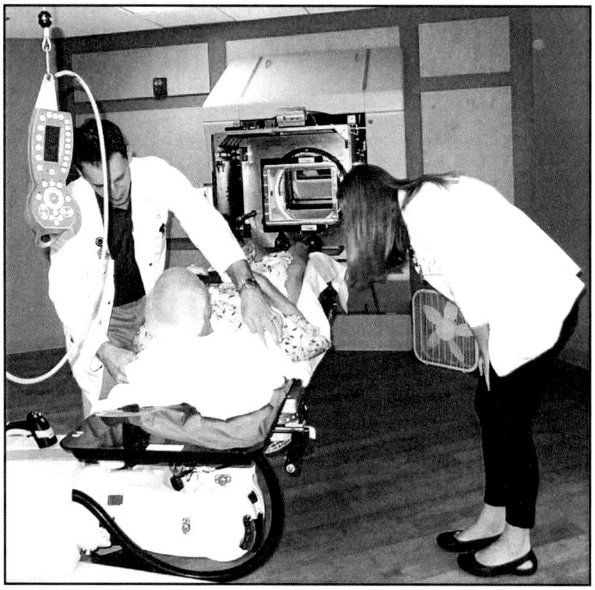

Here I am shown getting established on the table. It's flat and hard because any cushioning would introduce movement and thus imprecision. My legs rested in the cradle and my head on a soft pillow. Above, Kyle and Cortney lined me up.

When ready, I opened the door at the other end of the changing room, which leads to an inner hallway that serves two gantry rooms and one fixed beam room. Dramatic, circular, and futuristic-looking, the gantries can direct the beam from 360 degrees. Had I a hip replacement, metal, or other obstruction that prevented beaming from the sides, I would have been placed in a gantry room that beams from any angle.

A technician came for me and led me to the Autumn treatment room. After I entered the treatment room, one of the techs asked my birth date. "July 21, 1944." Then I walked over to the table, stepped up on the foot stool and swung my bare butt onto the white sheet. I snuggled my legs into the cradle, assuming the same position as during the original simulation.

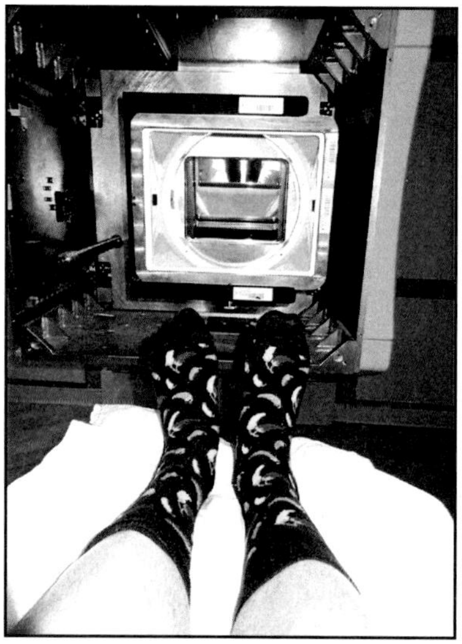

My treatment socks. The nozzle that emits the proton beams and X-rays can be seen in the background. My table turned so I was treated from each side.

The techs rolled up my gown from the sides and placed it on top of my legs, exposing my thighs but covering the genitals. One on each side of the table, the techs pulled on the sheet to move me in one direction or the other until the tattooed dots lined up in the laser crosshairs.

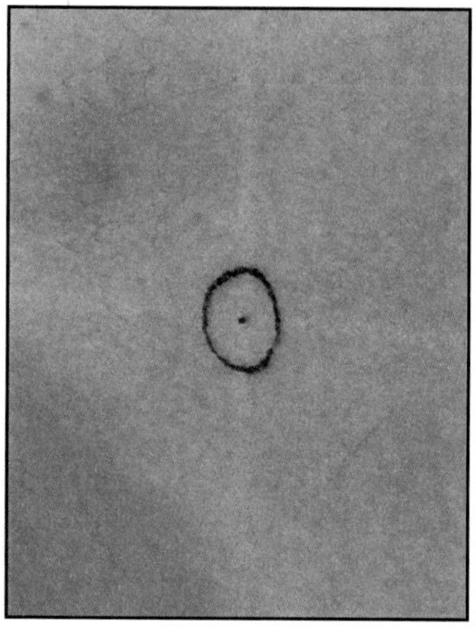

Lining up my tattooed dot. The tech added the circle with a ballpoint pen for the photo. They took numerous other photos for me, as well.

I stared up at ordinary soundproof ceiling tiles, less dramatic than a huge circular gantry. The X-ray equipment moved along a track cut into the ceiling. Out in the room, hand controls dangled from the ceiling. I've seen photos of many treatment rooms, all of which seem to have the same kind of hand controls. Recently I learned that IBA makes a cordless version now.

Once I was lined up, the X-ray equipment rolled into place above me. There were two flat plates, one above me and one to my side. Inside the nozzle, the X-ray tube slid into position.

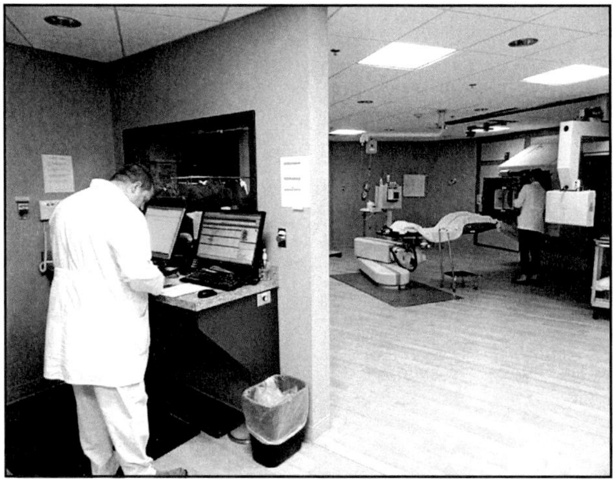

Treatment room. The techs go behind this wall during X-rays but completely out of the room during proton beam projection. Here Justin checks my details.

The technicians went behind a glassed-in area across the room to click the X-ray button. The horizontal X-ray came from the nozzle to the plate at my side, whereas the vertical X-ray came up from the floor and through the carbon fiber table to the plate above me.

The technicians had three screens in front of them: On the right, my original CT scan from the simulation; on the left, the digital X-ray just taken. The middle screen superimposed both images, which had to line up exactly.

The next image shows three areas with colored lines—one red, one green and one blue—called the "grapes." The three fiducials must fall within their respective grapes in both directions. Sometimes, to accomplish that, the computer adjusts the table position, thereby assuring precision within two millimeters variation (the thickness of a twenty-five cent coin).

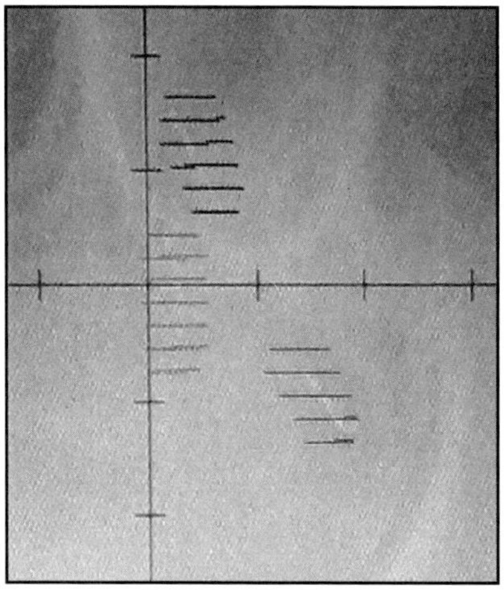

Two views of my three fiducial markers (two straight and one bent) which will remain inside of me for life. The grapes (left) are different colors.

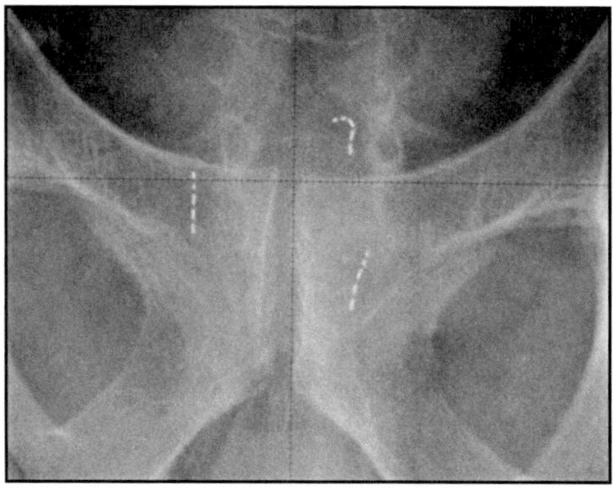

Satisfied with my positioning, the technicians returned, rolled away the X-ray equipment and said "Here we go." I stayed very still and didn't move an iota. To occupy my hands, I held a round rubber circle called the steering wheel over my chest with both hands. They then used a handheld barcode scanner and scanned barcodes on my table, my leg cradle, the nozzle, the degrader, everything (six or seven items). If anything was out of order, the proton equipment would not function, yet another check to assure accuracy.

A bell sounded, meaning everyone must leave the room (except me, of course). The techs exited by the same doorway through which we entered earlier. Protective doors closed first. Then a massive 60,000 pound (thirty-ton) door five feet thick, made of very dense concrete, rolled closed, half from each side. The walls are even thicker, giving protection from errant neutrons. From their control room, the techs kept on eye on me in their monitors.

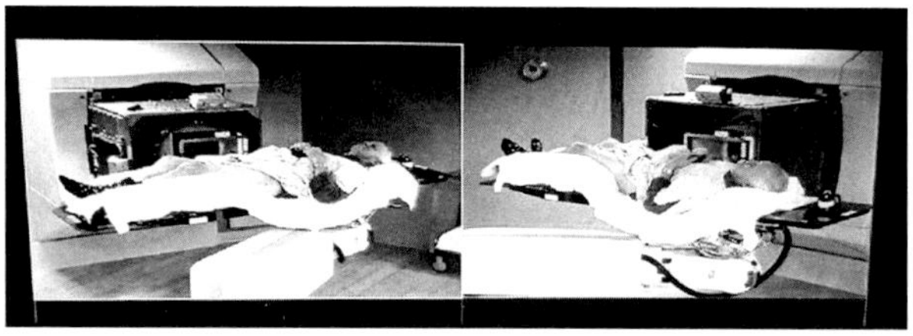

The techs' view of me in the monitor from behind the concrete walls and doors while I received my protons. The cameras showed two views.

I find the above photo very extraordinary. I know of no other book that shows proton therapy so explicitly. After the techs pressed the button, we waited our turn for the proton beam. More about the technology later. Computers controlled everything automatically. Sometimes the beam came right away, other times we waited a few minutes for it to finish its magic in one of the other treatment rooms.

Once it started, the beam scanned the prostate in sixteen layers. For each layer, the magnets made a slight mechanical growl. They reminded me of a scene in *Greystoke: The Legend of Tarzan, Lord of the Apes*, in which Tarzan, in England, goes up behind a woman sitting at the dinner table and makes the low, guttural sound of a lion, very primitive and dramatic. I saw the equipment like that lion, with the protons streaming in for the kill, disrupting the DNA of the cancer cells.

The protons completed their task in less than a minute. The door opened and the technicians reappeared, using the hand controls to turn my table around to expose my other side to the nozzle. We repeated the same procedure, taking the X-rays, merging the images, leaving the room, etc.

The rather extensive cancer in my prostate may have crept outside of the gland into the surrounding areas, even though not visible in the MRI scan. After seventeen treatments, the dose pattern changed to include my seminal vesicles and lymph nodes (a wider target). This protocol lasted until the end of my treatment. The same total dose was spread out more. I noticed a difference in the sound of the machine, longer and shorter adjustments totaling thirty-two layers. The shortest was just a little blip, whereas the longest growled for more than a second.

Finished, the techs returned, put my table back to the middle position, pulled my gown back over my legs and put down a little step stool to help me get off the table. Being in good shape, I popped right up and off. Apparently, some patients have a harder time. Typically, the whole process took fifteen to twenty minutes. I never felt hurried. After weeks together we got to know each other quite well, asking about the weekend or commenting on local football games. In my case, I took photos or gave my camera to the techs to do the same. I asked many questions about the procedures in order to understand and be able to explain it myself. Their answers reflected a deep knowledge of the system and its technical requirements, as well as the importance of precision.

Usually two techs attended me, sometimes three, depending on the length of the work day which in turn reflected the level of capacity at which they were operating. In 2018, two more treatment rooms became operational using revolutionary new equipment produced by ProNova, a sister company to Provision located in nearby Alcoa, Tennessee.

At the point when I was turned to treat the second side, one of the techs went into the lobby to bring in the next patient, to Autumn Changing Room Two. When I finished, they led me back to my changing room, Autumn One.

After we said our good-byes at the door, the tech stepped over to the adjacent changing room and accompanied that patient back to the treatment room. The goal was to keep the equipment in operation with the least amount of delay between patients. I followed this procedure thirty-nine times.

This timeline gives a visual idea of my daily schedule.

DAILY TIMELINE

6:00 a.m.	Arise
7:00	Breakfast
8:15	Leave home
9:15	Fitness center
10:15	Treatment
11:00	↑
Noon	
1:00 p.m.	
2:00	
3:00	
4:00	Free time
5:00	
6:00	
7:00	
8:00	
9:00	
10:00	↓

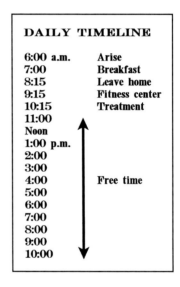

Notice how much free time we had. In his presentations, Robert Marckini illustrates what people think happens to proton patients by showing a slide of Frankenstein's monster strapped to a table. Then he shows them what actually takes place, with pictures of him playing golf every day. How true.

CHAPTER 7 SIDE EFFECTS

On Wednesdays I saw my doctor. After my treatment, I went to the small library area at the bottom of the stairs, took a clipboard and filled out the required form. I checked a series of boxes to self-report my condition. Here are my answers for day 17 and day 39

	Answer day (17)	*Answer day (39)*
Performance status (activity ability)	*Fully active*	*Fully active*
Fatigue level since starting treatment	*None*	*None*
Increase in urinary frequency	*Present**	*Present**
Urinary urgency	*Present**	*Present**
Urinary incontinence	*None*	*None*
Urinary tract pain (burning when urinating)	*None*	*None*
Hematuria (blood in urine)	*None*	*None*
Urinary retention	*None*	*None*
Diarrhea	*None*	*None*
Proctitis (rectal inflammation)	*None*	*None*
Abdominal pain	*None*	*None*
Fecal incontinence	*None*	*None*
Rectal hemorrhage	*None*	*None*
Radiation dermatitis	*None*	*None*
Unusual/excessive sweating	*None*	*None*
Medications used for symptoms	*None*	*Flomax*
Are you on testosterone blocking therapy	*No*	*No*

**Three choices: None, present, or limiting. This doesn't seem very descriptive of the most common side effect.*

The category "urinary retention" scared me the most. After "none" no good choices existed, such as "catheter placement" and "elected operative or radiologic intervention." Whew. These details got entered into a computer but won't be analyzed until they accumulate five years of data. Statistics of this kind will demonstrate the superiority of protons in limiting side effects.

The nurse came to the library and took me to record my weight and blood pressure. She asked a number of questions about how I was doing and whether I'd noticed any changes, typing the answers into her laptop. She had me show her my thighs to reveal any dermatitis from the X-rays. Even on the last day I never had any "sunburn," just a modest tan (barely visible on the photo below) that remains for months.

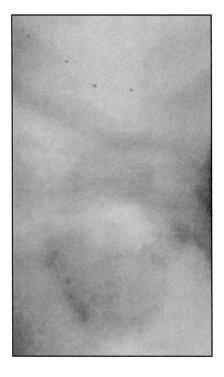

In a few minutes Dr. Fagundes came in. He looked at the form and my numbers, then asked if I had any questions. I reported that my urine flow was getting quite weak. He suggested I take Flomax, which is quite commonly used among patients here. I expressed concern over side effects, but he assured me it would be a low dose for a short time.

These relevant passages about side effects come from my journal (hence the purple color).

This afternoon while in Kohl's looking at gym clothes a sudden almost overwhelming urge to pee arose. I knew it wasn't real, not having a full bladder. It must be a side effect from the treatments (nine so far). I tightened my sphincter muscles until the feeling went away. Ten minutes later, it happened again, which I again thwarted. After ten more minutes, without the urge, I went to the restroom, feeling I had relieved myself on my own terms. This is far too early to be having side effects.

* * *

Today was not one of my better days. It was treatment #13, meaning I'm now one-third of the way. Over the weekend I noticed my urine stream was getting pretty weak. I presume the problem is that the urethra gets inflamed, which causes swelling which restricts the flow. Today the stream is so weak as to hardly be functional. I stand and wait for about five seconds for urine to even start. I presume this means it isn't flowing from the bladder very easily. This is scary for me. I don't want to take Flowmax. The nutritionist said that Omega-3 helps counter inflammation, so I will increase my fish oil supplements to three a day. I will also start having more ginger. Frankly, my stream was a little weak when I first got here. I may also go to the Vitamin Shoppe and look for an anti-inflammation supplement.

* * *

This morning my urine did not come out in a stream, just little squirts. I checked out Flomax to see what I might be looking forward to. It can lower blood pressure (good) but in so doing make me dizzy, give me rhinitis (stuffy nose, as with allergies), affect my mental state, and even cause tooth problems. It works to increase the flow but not to help urgency, although they usually go together. Urgency results from inflammation, which can be helped by taking some Ibuprofen.

* * *

Yesterday was day #20, meaning I have nineteen treatments behind me and the same number ahead of me. The situation has become urgent. I have been getting up three times a night and have many false urgencies when out in the public. I rushed to the restroom at Trader Joe's only to find it occupied. I waited so long I started knocking on the door. The urge lessened and I had plenty of time.

Last evening, before bedtime, I finally took a Flomax. Wow, it worked immediately. I got up only once during the night.

* * *

I've been a week now on Flomax. No side effects yet. This morning I was constipated, such that I did a Fleet enema. I've got it down now, quick and easy. I lie on my back on the bathroom floor and climb my feet up the wall to raise my butt in the air. Insert. Squeeze. Remove. Wait. Kaboom. If my constipation was a side effect, it never returned.

That was the last Fleet enema for the rest of my treatments. I used to make fun of the Flomax commercials which showed several old guys in a boat fishing. In my rewriting of the story, I have the guy taking Flomax stand up, get dizzy, and fall overboard. Flomax is made from tamsulosin, which is an alpha-blocker that relaxes the muscles in the prostate and bladder neck, making it easier for urine to flow. The pharmacist tells me it has been around for decades and has shown to be well tolerated.

The day after I started taking it, my symptoms improved. Not greatly, but enough. I felt remarkably strong and healthy during my treatments; urination was the only issue. With that issue out of the way, I felt like I was on vacation. Someone actually invented the term *radiation vacation*.

I asked other men about their side effects. One man taking both hormones and Flomax told me he was struggling. I didn't ask him to go into detail. Others made statements like, "Oh, there have been a few things, but very tolerable and better than the alternatives." Some difficulties result from the patient being in relatively poor condition upon arrival, with unhealthy lifestyles or diabetes or obesity.

I have completed twenty-seven treatments now, with twelve more to go. Still no more side effects. The Flomax is doing its job. No dermatitis from the radiation. No fatigue, although that's hard to say, as I have been experiencing some insomnia, a possible side effect of Flomax. I spend eight hours in bed to get five or six hours of sleep. Plus my afternoon nap, which sometimes extends well past the intended fifteen minutes.

I was told that proton beam therapy would continue to work for months, well after leaving Knoxville. There have been instances of rectal bleeding six months after treatment stopped. Apparently the weakened cancer cells take a while to expire. I continued taking Flomax until mid-December. By then, my flow surpassed the level when I first arrived in Knoxville. Now almost two years later, I have no side effects.

Back to San Antonio, I felt great. I'd just had two months of good diet, exercise, and a restful schedule, the benefits of a relaxing vacation. A friend who came over to welcome us home commented, "You still have your hair, or did it grow back?" He didn't understand my treatment. In fact, no one does. Over and over I tell my story.

I will monitor my PSA levels for the rest of my life. I met a man at one of my lectures whose PSA after his prostatectomy was 4.0. That meant the surgeon missed some of the cancer. Eighteen years later, he still takes hormones. Here are two stories told to me at Provision.

GEORGE'S STORY

George chose surgery even though only three of eighteen cores contained cancer. Aware of alternatives, he liked the idea of getting the diseased prostate out of his body. Other modalities make it inert or disable the cancer cells, but leave the prostate in place. He wanted it out of there. He recovered quickly, going back to the office part time as soon as the catheter was removed. Despite fatigue, he went on with his life. That sounded good until I learned more of the details. He did indeed lose sexual function, plus he had to endure another surgery for a complication that arose from the first surgery, the nature of which I didn't understand but it had something to do with intestines. Unfortunately, that remedial surgery didn't do the job; a third operation was required to remedy the problem.

KEN'S STORY

This story has a happy ending. Ken's urologist sent him to Dr. Busch at Diagnostic Radiology Consultants in Chattanooga for diagnosis. The 3-tesla MRI showed several lesions (tumors) in the prostate, which he estimated to be Gleason 7. That would seem to be enough to proceed with treatment, but not so fast. For insurance coverage, you must have a verifiable diagnosis to confirm the cancer, rather than have the "opinion" of someone interpreting a scan. So, Dr. Busch did a biopsy of only four cores, directed exactly to where the MRI located the cancer. The cores were all positive, satisfying the insurance company. The doctor then told Ken to go directly to Knoxville and Provision, which he did, very shortly receiving proton therapy.

I met a man to whom I described my excellent noninvasive treatment. He looked glum, hung his head and said, "I had surgery. I didn't know about protons." In my zeal to get out the word, I'll have to be sympathetic to those who never had the good fortune to find proton therapy.

Two weeks after arriving at Provision, I was sitting in a patient consulting room, madly scribbling down historical details about Provision being supplied by Nancy Howard, Vice President of Marketing and Public Relations. I told her my story, including the proposed date of September 14th for surgery. She looked at me and said, "That's today."

I was stunned. Riding back to our cottage I was lost in my thoughts. My mind was full of the contrast between surgery and proton beam therapy and the various directions in which my life could have gone. Once at our cottage, I looked up the post-surgery instructions the surgeon gave me. They included the following:

- *A small amount of bloody leakage from the wound is acceptable.*
- *It's okay to remove the catheter collection bag during showers.*
- *If the catheter falls out, call the surgeon immediately.*
- *Swelling and bruising of the scrotum should improve within fourteen days.*
- *To alleviate swelling, elevate the scrotum while sitting.*
- *Don't do any enemas, as they may damage the new connection between the bladder and urethra (hooked together after the prostate is removed from between them).*
- *Four weeks after surgery you can do relatively strenuous activities.*
- *Bring a urinary pad when the catheter is removed.*
- *Urinary control may not be regained for several months, fully, up to a year.*
- *You will leak more when standing up, moving, coughing, or laughing.*
- *Having removed the nerves, erections will no longer be possible.*
- *Some men experience a mild penile shortening after surgery (I had heard one inch. Let's be frank, I don't have any length to spare).*
- *Report fevers over 101 degrees (could mean infection).*
- *Report severe abdominal, flank or chest pain (could be other complications).*
- *Report nausea or vomiting.*

At that very moment, I realized, nurses would have been wheeling me back to my hospital room, facing some of the above consequences. Instead, here the some of the things I did on September 14th. .

- *Took a walk on the lovely Dowell Springs Campus along the water course.*
- *Worked out in the well-equipped fitness center.*
- *Received my twenty-minute painless noninvasive proton treatment.*
- *Shopped at Whole Foods for supplies to fix healthy meals at our cozy rented cottage.*

- *Went out for dinner at Bonefish to avail ourselves of half-price bang bang shrimp.*
- *Watched several episodes of "Chopped" on the Food Channel.*
- *Wrote in my journal and typed out notes from the day's meeting.*
- Turned *in for the night with my Sweetie, enumerating, as we always do, things for which we were grateful. At the top of my list is always the blessing of having Linda in my life and that we were together in Knoxville, Tennessee.*

Whew. Quite a difference.

Often, in the evenings, I sat out on our back deck and watched the sky fade into dusk and then darkness. The stars began to pop out. The freight trains shook the ground, the tracks being only about three hundred yards away. I sat out in the mornings, too, and tried my hand at poetry. Other than lining up words in little rows I know very little about poetry. Here's one of my morning poems.

EVIDENCE

through slits between the blinds
I see orange and yellow
colors of fall swaying with abandon
I turn to Linda and remark
"it's really windy out there"
even though I can't feel or
hear the wind I only see
the results of its action
on the visible trees in my yard

I think of those invisible protons
swirled pushed and pulled
by magnets then scanned to
their target in my prostate
this could be a complete hoax
and I would never know except
for the visible result of
going back to my excellent life
and many more happy years
with my Sweetie
my PSA barely evident

That prediction has proved to be the case. Yet, things are different now. I give special attention to any bodily issues or sensations. What was that pain in my groin? Always expecting the best, I remain vigilant should my health change. This typifies all cancer survivors. Almost two years out, I can tell you emphatically, so far, so good.

CHAPTER 8 GRADUATION

We arrived in Knoxville early afternoon of August 31, 2016. We left late morning on November 1, 2016, ecstatic. That September and October will always remain with me.

On my last day we arrived a little early and sat at our usual table. I had come to know a woman whose appearance caused me to make some false assumptions. Her white hair and demeanor made her appear elderly. She sat and crocheted, completing a poncho and other projects. She accompanied a man being treated for esophageal cancer.

Talking with the woman, I discovered she was quite sharp, her voice strong with its Tennessee accent. On the morning of my graduation, she went over to the piano and started to play some hymns. She missed a few notes at first, perhaps from stiff fingers, but after ten minutes she got warmed up. She shifted into gospel music with quite a swing to it. Subtly, employees wandered out from the back to look and see who was playing so well.

She really tickled those keys, playing everything from memory. I suspect she once accompanied a gospel choir. She certainly took me by surprise and set a joyous tone for the completion of my treatments.

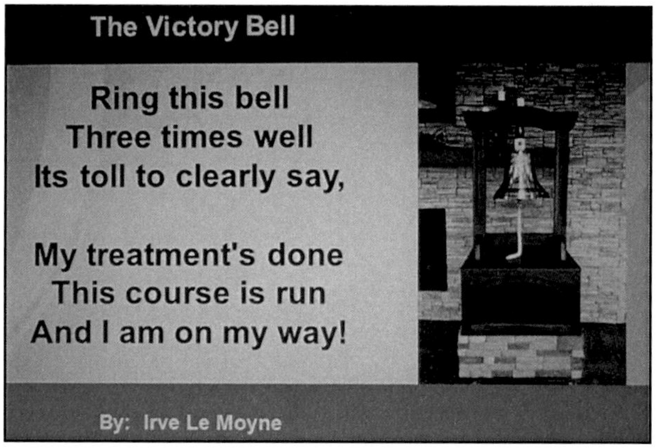
The Victory Bell
Ring this bell
Three times well
Its toll to clearly say,
My treatment's done
This course is run
And I am on my way!
By: Irve Le Moyne

According to Provision, the custom of ringing a bell started in 1996 when Navy admiral Irve LeMoyne neared the end of his cancer treatment. He told the doctor he wanted to ring a bell when the job was done, which is a Navy tradition. I became familiar with a similar ceremony at Wings Clinic in Memphis, Tennessee when I built for them a single-path labyrinth designed to be walked as a form of meditation. They had a local sculptor build a tower with a bell. After finishing chemotherapy, the patients would get a bouquet of yellow balloons, walk the labyrinth, and then ring the bell to mark their return to their normal lives.

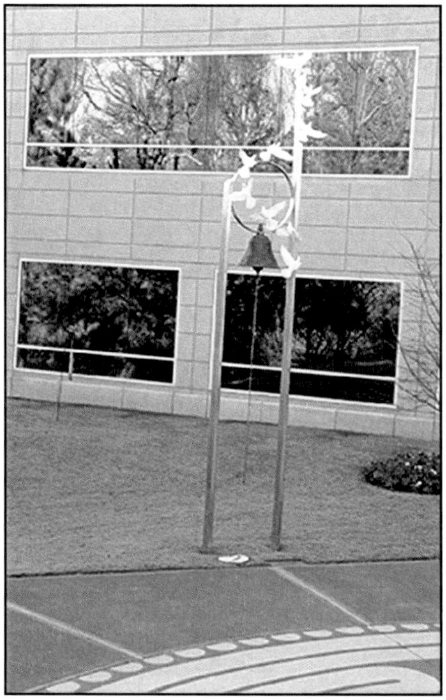

The ceremonial bell at Wings Clinic. The doves, to me, represent the freeing of the spirit after the fear and uncertainty of one's cancer journey. Note the edge of the labyrinth in the foreground.

Patients at Provision devised their own ceremonies, which differed considerably from person to person. One man just walked, rang the bell three times very quickly, and then walked away. No big deal. Usually, those of us in the lobby at the time gathered around. More than once a large group of friends and family members came for the event. The graduates usually give a short talk, without exception praising the staff, the setting, and the treatment. Some sing the doxology or other hymns.

Each time I attended a graduation, I was aware that one day it would finally be my turn to stand there. One man, treated for a brain tumor, kept as a souvenir the mask he wore during treatment. The mask held his head immobile while receiving the protons. He, like many others, became emotional, the ceremony representing the end of a very terrifying journey with cancer and the new freedom to return home to a normal life and future despite seemingly impossible odds.

Another man told how he arrived expecting to endure a cold medical atmosphere. Instead, he found himself embraced by fellow patients and enveloped in the culture of care. Another man advised me, "Get the names and Facebook pages of everyone so you can stay in touch. We're all family now." One man rang the bell, said a few words, and rushed back to Myrtle Beach, South Carolina, as his homes and vehicles were in the path of approaching hurricane Matthew.

During my treatments I always wore my special hot pepper socks, which I thought were unique. Then I discovered that a man who called himself Krazy Kramer wore a different pair of fancy socks every day, leaving them behind in a big jar. He sent the following poem on a poster, along with photos of his socks:

I arrived alone and concerned.
My cancer was all I saw.
I'm leaving Provision with dozens
of friends, hundreds of laughs
and SO MANY funny stories!!!
I hope you ALL realize
how important you are to
each of us as we muddle
through our fractions.
Your smiles, kind words and
hugs are much more
powerful than any speeding protons.

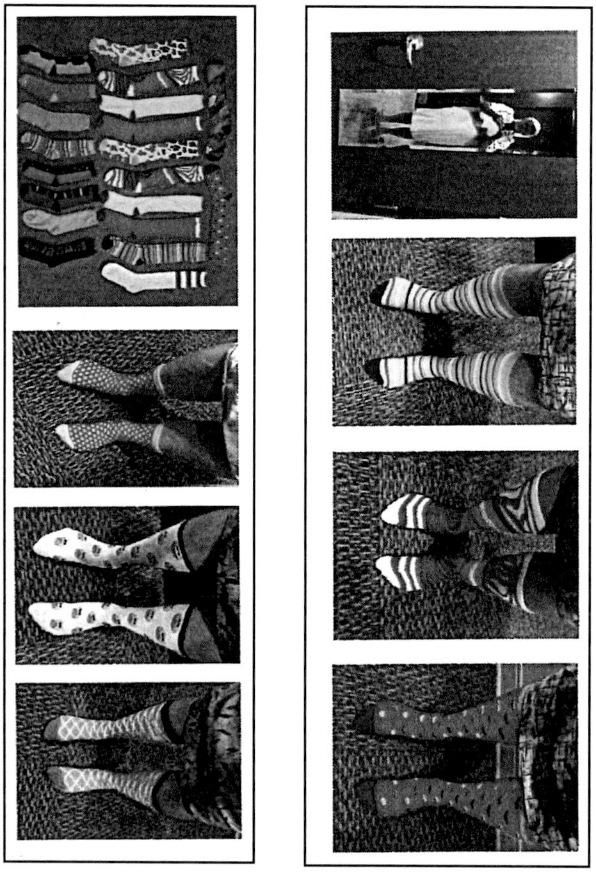

Kramer's colorful socks.

Early on I made a calendar with thirty-nine squares from September 8 to November 1 so I could cross off the treatment days. During my graduation ceremony, I took a fat brown felt tip marker and made a large "X" in the last remaining box (photo).

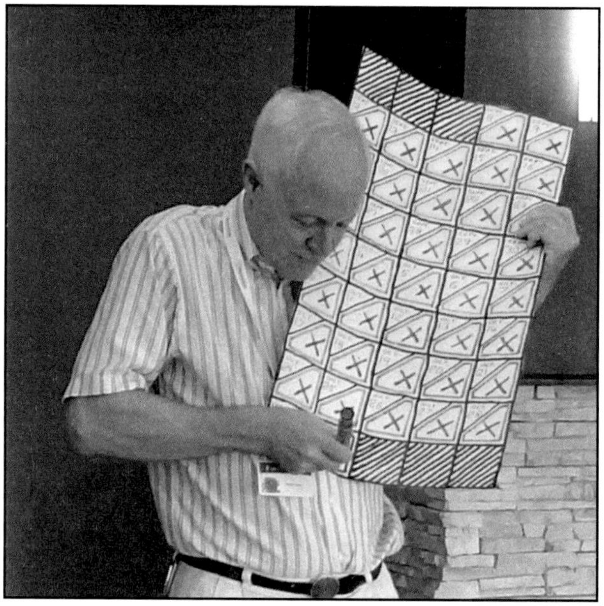

Not feeling much emotion (just relief) I spoke without getting teary except when I thanked Linda for being my support person. Finally the time comes to ring the victory bell.

Already packed and ready to go back to Texas, the car awaited us out in the parking lot. Elizabeth came over, clearly stalling for time. Finally, she gave me my pin and a certificate saying I was graduate number 1,232. Then, Samantha showed up. Yes! She was the first person I talked to at Provision and the one who answered my questions and told me about Medicare payments. She's the one who changed my life. We repeated the ceremony and this time Samantha gave me the pin and certificate.

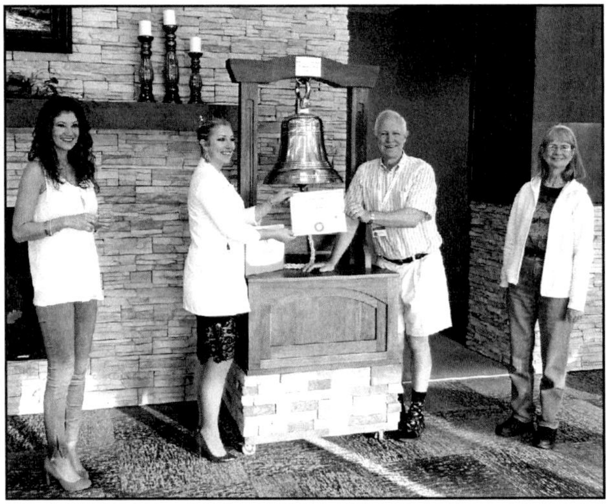

Elizabeth, Samantha, Robert, Linda.

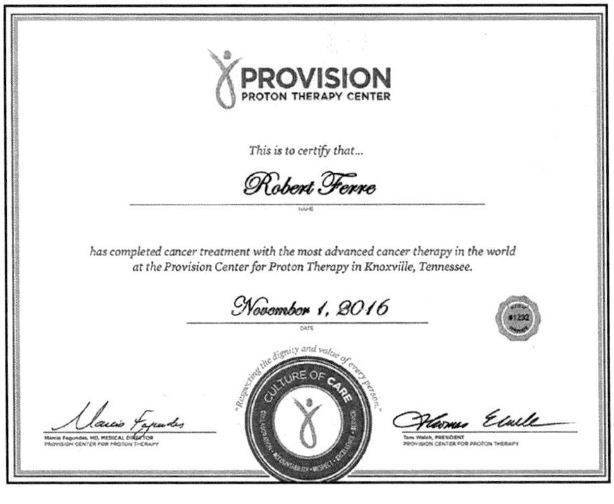

PROVISION
PROTON THERAPY CENTER

This is to certify that...

Robert Ferre

NAME

has completed cancer treatment with the most advanced cancer therapy in the world at the Provision Center for Proton Therapy in Knoxville, Tennessee.

November 1, 2016

DATE

"Respecting the dignity and value of every person."

CULTURE OF CARE

Marcio Fagundes, MD, MEDICAL DIRECTOR
PROVISION CENTER FOR PROTON THERAPY

Tom Welch, PRESIDENT
PROVISION CENTER FOR PROTON THERAPY

My certificate.

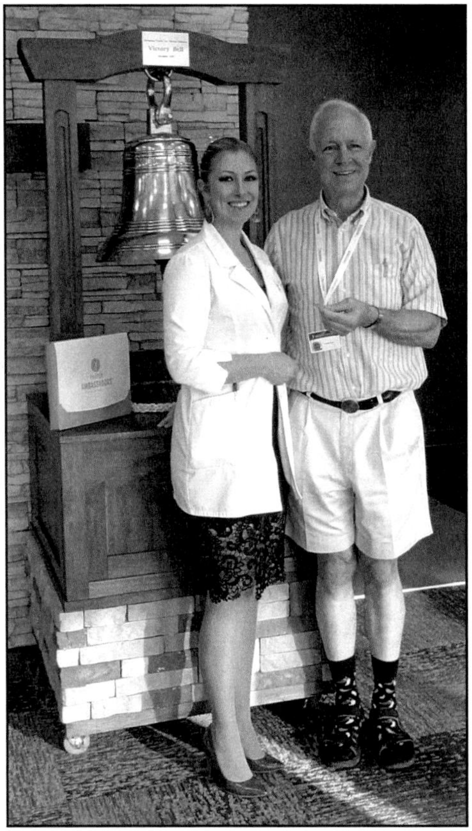

Samantha and me. I wore shorts to show off my special hot pepper treatment socks.

When the moment came to ring the bell, Linda and I did it together, as we had done with everything for the whole journey. One on each side, we slowly rang the bell three times.

After the ceremony we shook hands with our fellow patients and spouses. Sometimes the radiation techs come out, but my principal ones, Justin and Cortney, were busy. They're the true interface with Provision. Despite all of the technology and quality assurance and double checks, when it gets right down to it, human beings line me up and turn on the protons. The equipment, while impressive, is also cold and passive. Not so the staff.

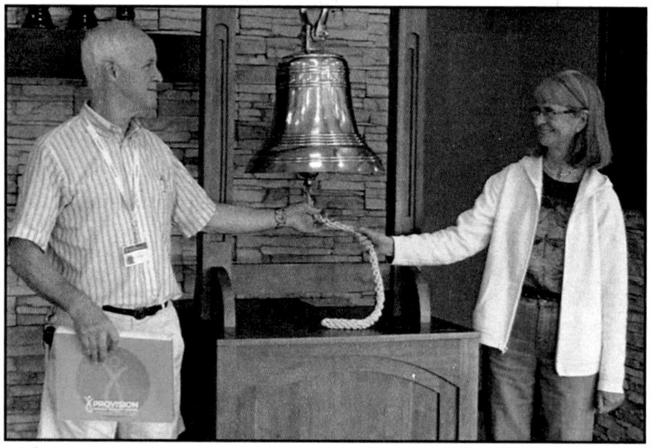

Linda and I ring the completion bell.

It took just minutes to get on Interstate 40 West and then Interstate 75 through Chattanooga. With no more dietary restrictions, I went crazy. The first and second days of driving I ate cruciferous vegetables galore (broccoli, Brussels sprouts, cauliflower). I had a big bowl of granola and lots of fruit for breakfast. I ordered grits, biscuits (gluten and all) and gravy (with sausage), cornbread and honey (yes, Cracker Barrel). I had beans. I wondered if my digestive system would object. Oh, yes, it sure did. I paid the price.

We visited friends in Houston for a day and night, finally reaching San Antonio on Friday, November 4, 2016. It was time to get on with our lives. And so we did (see photo on page 115).

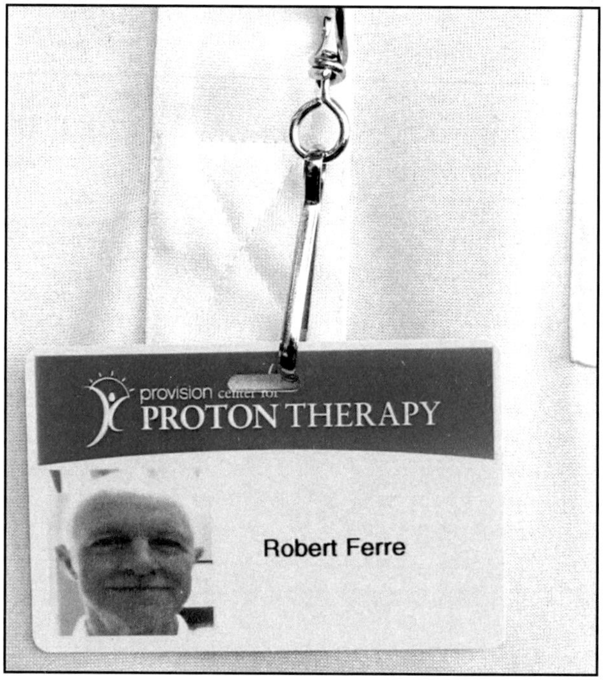

A souvenir that I would rather never have had. However, under the circumstances, it could hardly have been a better experience.

CHAPTER 9 THE PHYSICS OF PROTONS

Warning! This chapter may be a bit challenging for the nontechnical reader. Feel free to just look at the pictures as I give a quick overview of the technology.

Proton therapy requires a source of protons, an accelerator to increase their speed, a selection system to adjust the energy level, a magnet-controlled beam line to shape and transport the proton stream, a delivery system, and a positioning system to move the beam, the patient, or both. Got that?

Proton therapy is a form of radiation. I find that confusing because we must distinguish between the electromagnetic and particulate forms.

Electromagnetic radiation stretches across a wide spectrum, determined by wave length, part of which is visible light. The type of X-rays used for cancer treatment are pure energy, which can be quantized into discrete packets called photons.

Particulate radiation involves particles from the center of atoms, which differ from X-rays in that they have mass. The protons used in prostate cancer therapy come from the nuclei of hydrogen atoms (see drawing). Hydrogen represents the most common and stable element in the universe. Each atom has one electron and one proton. Protons can be derived from water or hydrogen gas. Provision uses hydrogen gas, which is zapped by an electric arc to destabilize the atoms. Magnets strip away the electrons and pull the protons into the cyclotron which accelerates them to two-thirds the speed of light. As they gain speed, protons gain kinetic energy.

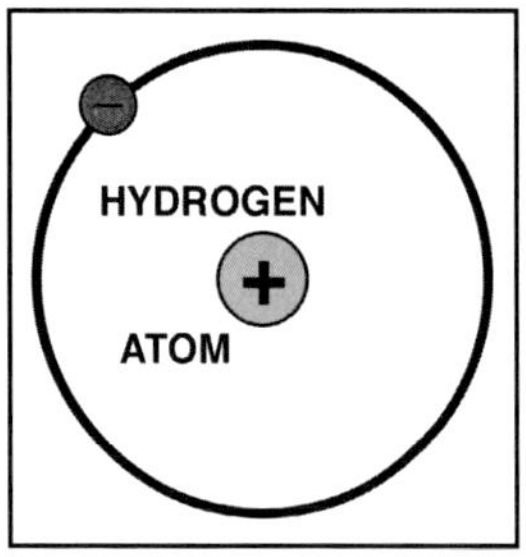

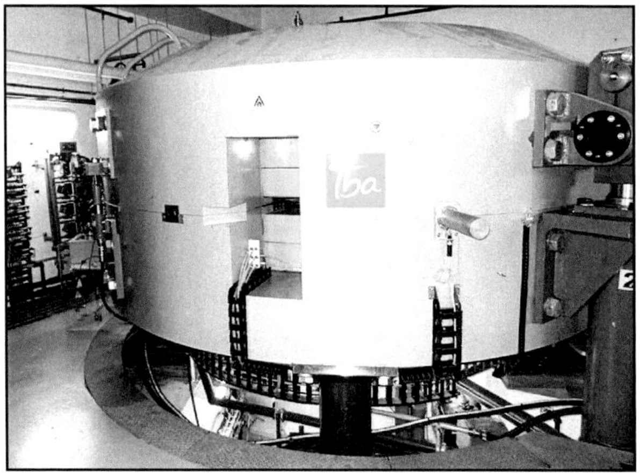

IBA Cyclotron comprising 220 tons of copper and iron.

One way of quantifying proton energy is in electron volts, eV, a million of which is written MeV. Protons at Provision can reach up to 250 MeV or as low as 70 MeV.

The cyclotron used in my treatment came from Ion Beam Applications, SA (IBA) and shipped all the way from Belgium.

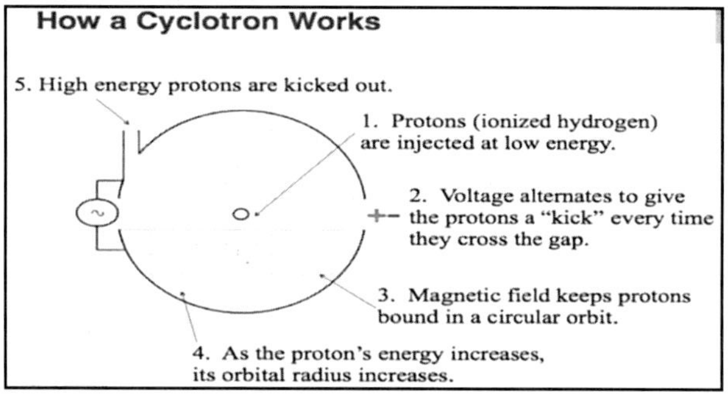
How a Cyclotron Works
5. High energy protons are kicked out.
1. Protons (ionized hydrogen) are injected at low energy.
2. Voltage alternates to give the protons a "kick" every time they cross the gap.
+−
3. Magnetic field keeps protons bound in a circular orbit.
4. As the proton's energy increases, its orbital radius increases.

Each time the proton passes through a gap in the cyclotron, it increases its energy 50,000 eV (thus, 200,000 eV per revolution, as there are four gaps). After 1,100 revolutions the proton reaches the desired energy of 220MeV. Those 1,100 revolutions take a very tiny fraction of a second, as does the rest of their trip to my prostate. (The protons would circumnavigate the earth five times in one second.)

The protons travel down a beam line within a vacuum (to keep them from contamination from ambient air) except for one place called the degrader. Since all of the protons are released from the cyclotron with the same energy, to vary that energy (and hence the distance the proton beam travels inside my prostate) requires an intervention in the form of the degrader. It looks like a wedge wrapped around a cylinder. Depending on the position of the wedge, the protons travel through more or less attenuating material.

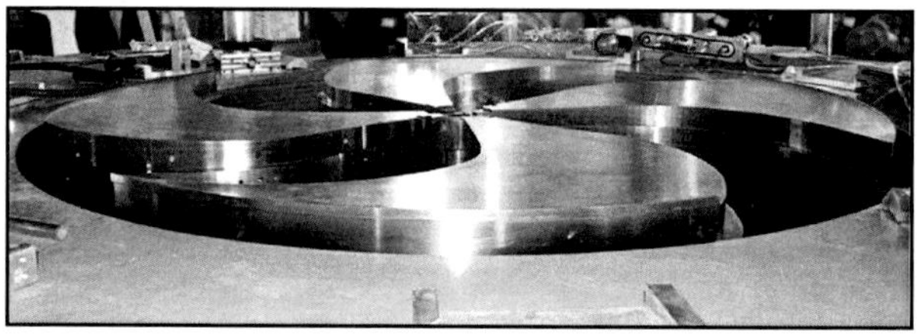

The inside of the cyclotron with the four gaps that accelerate the protons.

During my treatment, I heard the movement of the scanning magnets directing each layer of protons, followed by three or four seconds of silence while the degrader reduced the energy ever so slightly for the next layer of protons just proximal to (in front of) the previous layer. Thus, the prostate gets treated from its farthest point to the closest point.

Emerging from the degrader, the protons travel through a vacuum line in an organized beam shaped and controlled by magnets. Being positively charged, protons naturally repel each other (like the same poles of magnets), trying to spread out. If that happens, the protons get disorganized and become uncontrollable. To prevent this, strong magnets keep the protons together in an organized beam (hence, proton *beam* therapy).

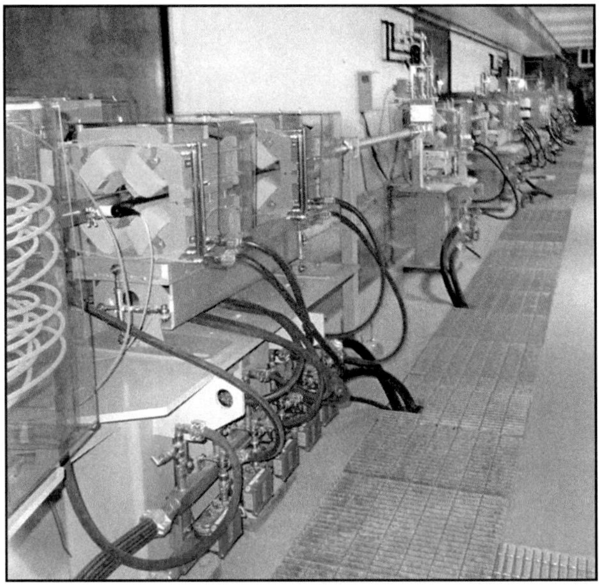

Above: The beam line, passing through numerous magnets. Below: IBA control room.

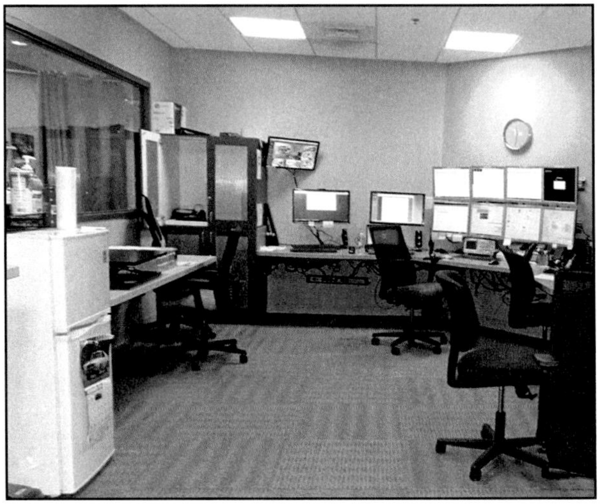

The quality and consistency of the beam are of the utmost importance. Twenty-four hours a day a team of a dozen trained engineers from IBA monitor and test the beam. Every aspect of the technology remains under constant observation.

At 9:45 pm, when only the guard keeps watch over the empty lobby and a few therapists tie up loose ends at the end of a long day, they arrive—mostly young, jeans-clad, ready to do the behind-the-scenes, after-hours work that keeps Provision treating cancer patients.

Tonight's four-man night crew is among 12 total IBA employees responsible for the treatment gantries, cyclotron, and larger proton therapy system—manufactured by Belgium-based IBA—that make proton therapy possible. They work in three shifts, starting at 5:30 a.m. and 1:30 and 10:00 p.m., rotating crews every three weeks.

They are little seen behind the closed doors of their control room and in the bowels of the facility's equipment rooms, but the team is crucial to ensuring patients receive treatment on time and at the correct dose.

The above paragraphs are from the Provision website. Once, during my treatment, the sound of the magnets stopped for some thirty or forty seconds and then started again. When I asked the tech what caused that, he said the beam went out of calibration, as measured by three consecutive ion chambers at the treatment end of the beam line, which automatically shuts down the system to correct the adjustment. With the issue resolved, the treatment resumed. This was just one more check to make sure the protons did their work properly.

I interviewed Provision physicists for six hours, attended several lectures and watched YouTube videos, accumulating many pages of notes, some of it too technical to include here (gaussian curves, sigma, etc.). Perhaps the physicists will be amused when they read my simplified version and unscientific vocabulary.

Gates direct the protons to the appropriate treatment room. Switching between rooms in 2016 took about twenty seconds, but newer equipment is much faster. The same is true for the degrader, which will be located in each individual treatment room rather than next to the cyclotron.

To deliver the protons to the patient requires either a gantry, which turns around the patient, or a fixed beam, which stays in one place while the patient's position moves. Since prostates are easy to access from the side, I was in a fixed beam room.

To revolve the proton beam 360 degrees around the treatment table looks simple enough. The nozzle changes position with the push of a button. However, behind the wall turns a huge gantry, three stories tall, weighing anywhere from fifty to two hundred tons, all of which turns along with the nozzle. Bending the beam takes strong magnets, which are very heavy and need counterweights. That's the best explanation I can give for why the gantry needs to be so large.

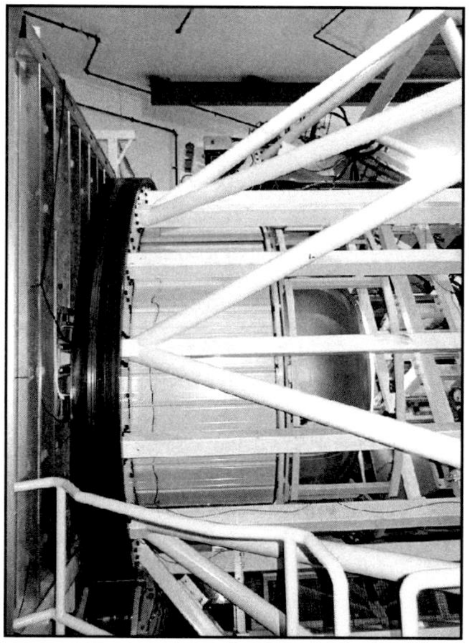

This gantry lies out of sight behind the wall at Provision. The whole structure turns along with the nozzle. While I realize the difficulty in bending proton beams, I can't explain the huge size of the gantry.

On the tour of the facility I saw the Provision gantries but couldn't get far enough away to take a full photo.

Once the beam reaches the treatment room, it must be directed and controlled to best serve its purpose. The latest technology for doing this is pencil beam scanning (PBS), which gets its name from delivering spots about the same circumference as a pencil. The original technology involves uniform double-scattering, which is still widely in use.

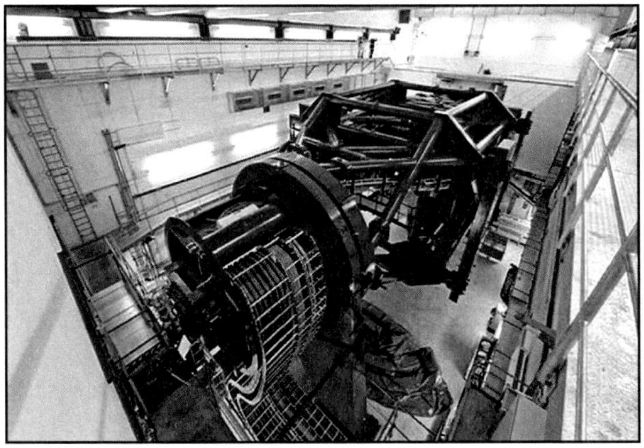

Here is a gantry at Heidelberg University in Germany. Behind the wall on the left is the treatment room. The circular area next to the wall is the tunnel in which the patient lies. When the nozzle moves, the entire gantry turns. (Used with permission. For information see https://www.heidelberg-university-hospital.com/diseases-treatments/tumor-diseases/proton-therapy-and-carbon-ion-therapy/)

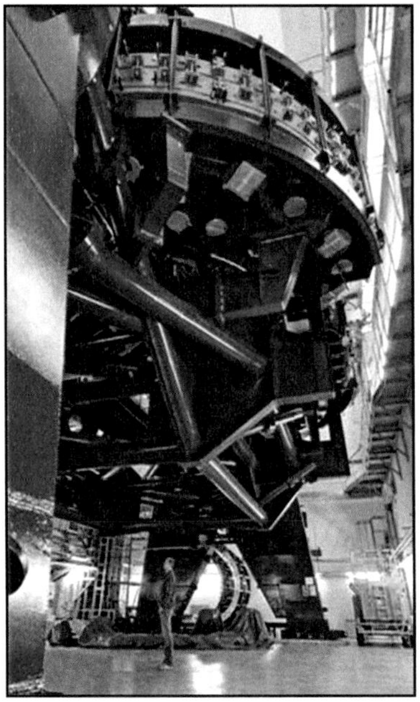

Also at Heidelberg University is this gigantic gantry for utilizing carbon ions, which may be even more effective than protons. I believe it is the only one of its kind in the world. Notice the person standing beneath it.

As previously mentioned, once the proton beam reaches the patient, it must be effectively directed to the target. Uniform scanning projects the protons in a plane, basically rectangular. The width depends on the degree of scattering, usually involving two steps (hence double-scattering). The beam is conformed to the shape of the prostate by using an aperture through which the beam passes, thereby assuming the shape of the prostate. Each one must be custom made, often of brass, sometimes of other materials. After completing treatment, the patient keeps the aperture as a unique souvenir paper weight.

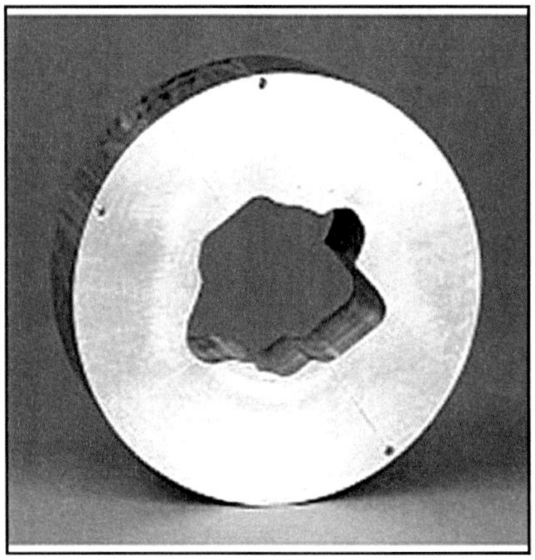

An aperture made of brass. The opening conforms the beam to the shape of the prostate being treated.

PBS works differently than uniform double-scattering, a critically important difference that opens up a world of new possibilities. It forms a series of layers by laying down rows of overlapping spots.

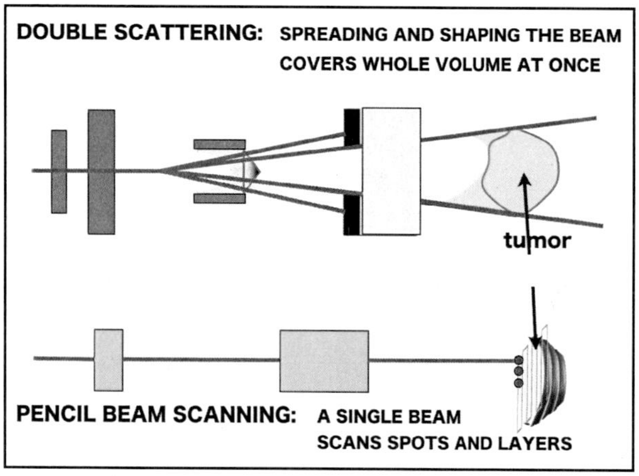

Two methods for delivering protons.

Think of scattered protons as covering a whole surface and pencil beam as hitting a series of specific spots. Note the greater simplicity of PBS, mechanically. Double-Scattering can treat around twenty percent of all cancers. PBS, on the other hand, can treat eighty percent of all cancers, a huge increase.

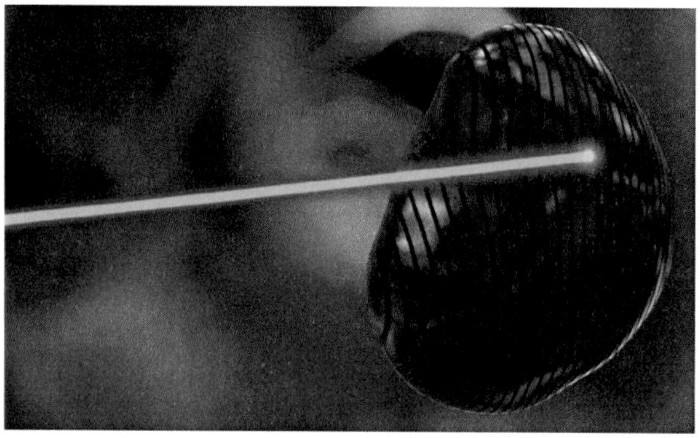

Three-dimensional illustration of pencil beam scanning provided courtesy of IBA. They also have a video showing how it scans layer by layer.

Just before reaching me the proton beam passed through a range shifter, which was a removable rectangular screen that slid into the front of the snout at the end of the nozzle adjacent to the treatment table. They had two such screens, one four centimeters (called a "forty," referring to millimeters) and the other seven and one-half centimeters (a "seventy-five"). I required the forty. Four centimeters equals about one and one-half inches. If you line up two pennies side by side, they measure about one and one-half inches across.

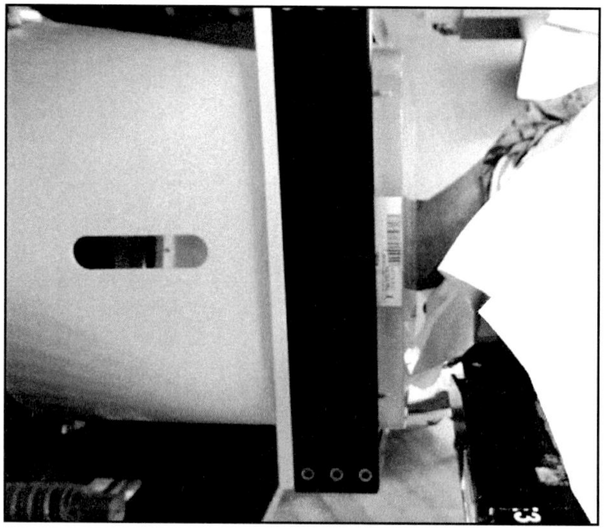

This photo shows me on the treatment table, taken from down by my feet. My right arm hangs off the table. You can see the close proximity of the snout to my thigh. Note the laser beam that indicates proper alignment. The range shifter screen sits on the front of the snout, right next to my arm, with a bar code to identify it.

The nomenclature doesn't refer to the thickness of the range shifter screen, but rather, the amount the screen attenuates (slows down) the protons. The degrader near the cyclotron also makes adjustments, as previously explained. As with all the components for each individual patient in the treatment room, the techs scan the barcodes to confirm they have the one designated for that patient.

When the beam finally reaches the patient on the treatment table, there remains one more element, namely, the computer-controlled maneuverability of the table itself. As described in the chapter about my treatment, X-rays confirm that the final alignment matches the original simulation. Finally, the protons do their work, taking no more than a minute or so. Multiplied by my thirty-nine treatments they added up to about an hour under the beam. (That would be a great book title).

Pencil beam scanning is such an exciting development that I wrote a second book about the subject, *Proton Therapy: Revolutionary Treatment for 80% of ALL Cancers.*

So there you have it, the story of protons starting as hydrogen gas, ionized, accelerated, degraded, beamed, rotated (in some cases, but not mine), examined, range shifted, and finally scanned in successive layers, all to treat my prostate cancer. Many people to whom I talk have no idea what protons even are, much less how they can be used medically. In the next chapter I explain where this extraordinary technology originated.

CHAPTER 10 HISTORY

Proton beams behave according to the unique characteristics of hydrogen ions. Specifically, they deposit their energy in a sudden burst at the end of their journey, called the Bragg Peak —or sometimes, Bragg's Peak, as illustrated in the chapter on dosimetry (p. 73).

William Henry Bragg, professor of physics and mathematics at Adelaide University in Australia from 1896 to 1909, wrote about this phenomenon more than a century ago. Naming this phenomenon after him gives him his due recognition. Little could he have imagined proton therapy today. He might even smile.

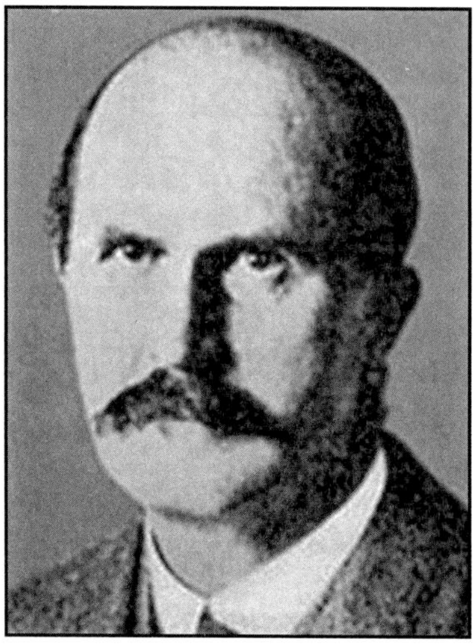

Sir William Henry Bragg

In 1943, a young physicist at Princeton, Robert Wilson, joined the efforts in Los Alamos, New Mexico, for the ultra-secret Manhattan Project to develop a nuclear weapon. Still in his twenties, he became the youngest group leader, using a cyclotron shipped to Los Alamos from Harvard University to study measurements of the neutron cross section of plutonium.

After Germany surrendered, Wilson felt research should stop, but it continued until the United States dropped two nuclear bombs on Japan. Thereafter, Wilson lobbied strongly for international control of nuclear weapons. The National Association for Proton Therapy gives this history:

After the end of the Second World War, building on discoveries made during work on the Manhattan Project and other activities, a group of scientists and physicists developed particle accelerators of much higher energy and began applying what they had learned to help benefit mankind. They focused on the application of nuclear medicine for diagnostic purposes and the treatment of certain diseases. One particularly interesting possibility had to do with improving the treatment of cancerous tumors, especially those previously unreachable or not treatable without inducing significant damage to healthy surrounding tissues. Wilson helped design a new 150 MeV cyclotron for Harvard to replace the one sent to New Mexico and accepted an appointment as associate professor. Regretting his part in the creation of such great destruction he decided to turn his knowledge to medical research in order to benefit humanity rather than destroying it.

At Harvard in 1946, Wilson published a seminal paper, "Radiological Use of Fast Protons," which founded the field of proton therapy. He proposed using accelerator-produced beams of protons to treat deep-seated tumors in humans. In that paper, he explained the biophysical rationale for proton therapy as well as the key engineering techniques of beam delivery. In 1954, the first human was treated with proton beams at the Lawrence Berkeley Laboratory.

In 1962, specialized radiosurgical proton treatments commenced at the Harvard Cyclotron Laboratory, followed in the mid-1970s by treatments for ocular cancers and larger tumors. Physicists at Harvard, collaborating with clinical colleagues, developed much of the physics and technology needed to treat patients with proton beams safely and effectively. Remarkably, the research and development program at Harvard continued for more than forty years. From Harvard Wilson went to Cornell and then to be director of the Fermi National Accelerator Laboratory (named after Enrico Fermi, usually shortened to Fermilab) near Chicago, Illinois where he had a direct role in designing the facility. The following comes from Fermilab's website:

Wilson had studied sculpture at the Academia de Belle Arti di Fienze in Florence, Italy, while on sabbatical in 1961, and he wanted Fermilab to be an appealing place to work, believing that external harmony would encourage internal harmony as well, and labored personally to keep it from looking like a stereotypical "government lab," playing a key role in its design and architecture.

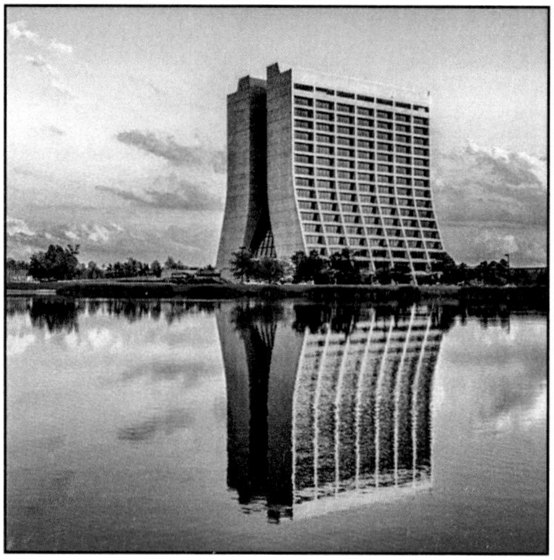

The building Wilson helped design.

Surrounding the facility was a restored prairie which served as home to a herd of American bison that started with Wilson bringing in a bull and four cows in 1969.

The site features ponds and Wilson's building, purposely reminiscent of Beauvais Cathedral in France. Fermilab also celebrates his role as a sculptor, featuring several of his works. In 1980 they renamed the central laboratory building Robert Rathbun Wilson Hall in his well deserved honor.

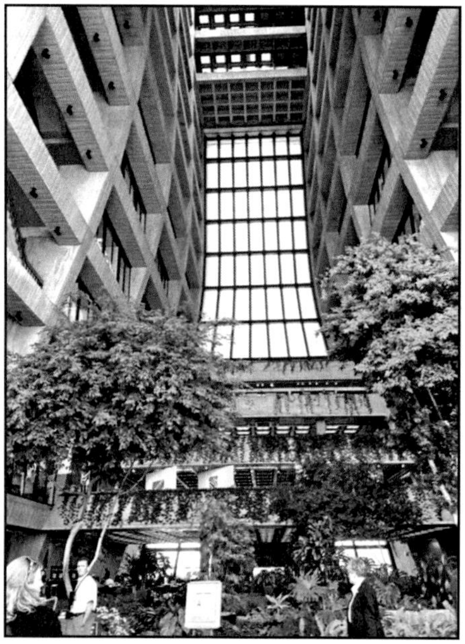

Above: The inside of the building shown on the previous page, designed to resemble Beauvais Cathedral, the tallest of the French Gothic cathedrals (below).

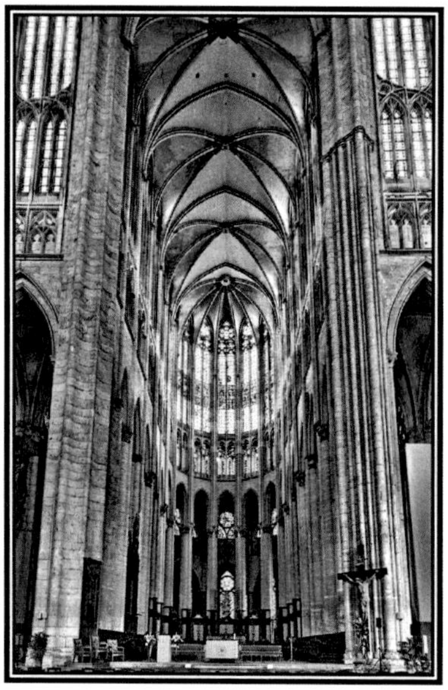

Wilson resigned as director of Fermilab in 1978 to protest what he felt was inadequate funding and support from the federal government. In the initial building stage, however, he had $250 million to work with. Construction came in on time and under budget.

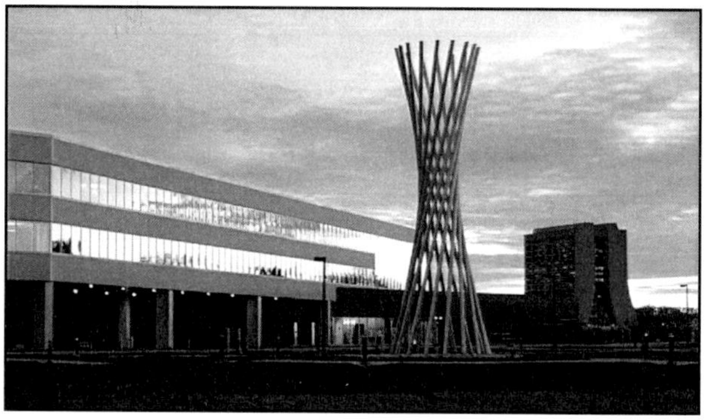

Fermilab buildings and Wilson's sculpture Tractricious.

In the meantime, technologies continued to advance, including accelerators, magnetically scanned beams, treatment planning systems, computed tomographic (CT) imaging, and magnetic resonance imaging (MRI).

The first treatments using protons could be performed only with access to accelerators, whether cyclotrons or synchrotrons, as at Berkeley Radiation Laboratory in 1954 and Uppsala, Sweden, in 1957. In 1961, Harvard and Massachusetts General Hospital jointly pursued proton therapy, refining and expanding these techniques over the next four decades while treating 9,116 patients before shutting down the cyclotron in 2002.

In 1989, the Clatterbridge Centre for Oncology in the United Kingdom became the world's first hospital-based proton therapy center using a low energy cyclotron for ocular tumors. A few years before, at Loma Linda University in California, the medical center sought someone to build a proton synchrotron and beam transport system. After considerable debate, the University dedicated $1,500,000 to the project. I consider that act of vision as the single most important step in the development of proton beam therapy. Several companies they approached turned down the challenge until they contacted Fermilab, the same facility founded by Robert Wilson.

Fermilab agreed to build the system, for which the cost and installation became so high the United States government finally came to the rescue with $25 million additional dollars. Dr. James M. Slater, a researcher in the Loma Linda University radiation department, promoted and oversaw the project. In 1990 they treated thc first patient at what was the first hospital-based proton treatment center in the United States. In 1994 the second and third gantries became operational.

In 2007 Loma Linda changed their name to the James M. Slater, MD, Proton Treatment and Research Center. In their twenty-five plus years of operation, they have treated more than twenty thousand cancer patients. Their courageous leadership led the way.

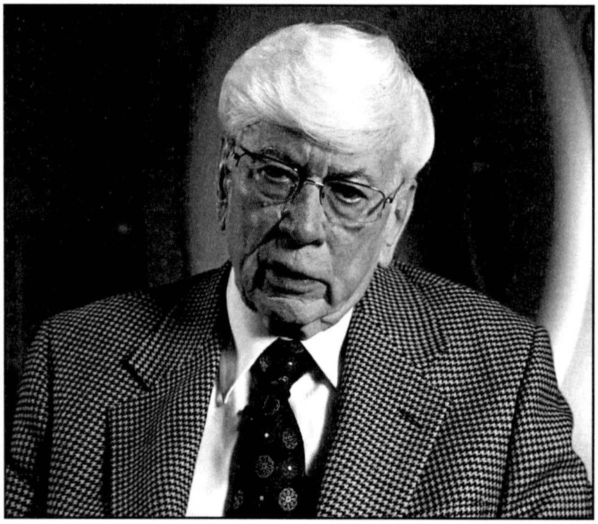

Dr. James M. Slater, MD.

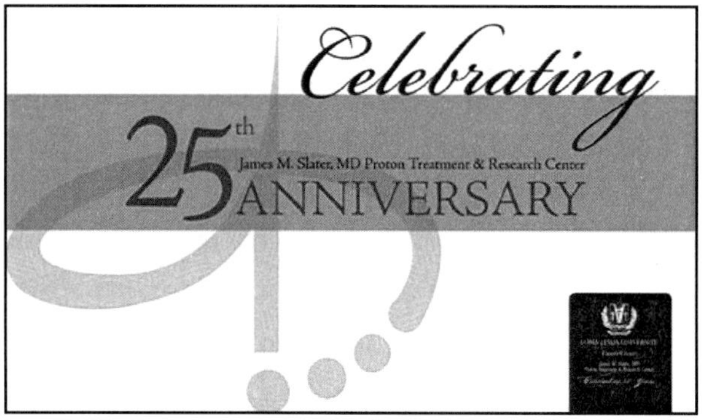

At the end of this book I have a list of proton treatment centers. It took thirteen years before the next full proton therapy center opened at Mass General Hospital in 2003. Three years later the third center opened at M. D. Anderson in Houston, Texas. Next came the University of Florida Proton Therapy Institute in Jacksonville, Florida, a nonprofit organization affiliated with the University of Florida College of Medicine and the University of Florida Shands Cancer Center. Their-five year study of results for proton therapy shows a success (non-recurrence) rate ranging from 98 to 99 percent.

It took two decades for the first five centers to open. In the past six years, twenty more centers have joined them, with sixteen more in the planning or building stages. As costs drop and demand increases, even more centers will open. In a growing number of cases, two cities have or will soon have two proton centers competing with each other. The state of Florida will have seven centers.

The growth of new centers has not been without controversy. Some still claim that the results do not sufficiently merit the enormous increase in cost. Within a few years, that will no longer be an issue. ProNova, a sister company of Provision, offers smaller and less expensive state-of-the-art systems. They consider the construction in Franklin, Tennessee (near Nashville) of the Proton CARES Proton Therapy Center to be their prototype for future centers.

How do they specifically apply this technology to determine the best dose of protons for each patient? The next chapter covers the important topic of dosimetry.

CHAPTER 11 DOSIMETRY

That someone could figure this out, design the equipment, construct a building to hold it, train technicians and keep it all running I find nothing short of miraculous. In my opinion, this may be the most important chapter in this book in that it describes exactly how the right number of protons are directed to the specific target to most effectively nutrilize the cancer without obliterating healthy tissue.

The book *Proton & Charged Particle Radiotherapy* states it like this.

> *The precision of dose distribution with charged particles means that radiation doses can be delivered to the tumor with less irradiation to the surrounding normal tissue and permits selective dose escalation to the tumor. Because higher radiation doses to the tumor increase the likelihood of sterilizing the tumor cells and because irradiation of less normal tissue and/or delivery of lower dose to the same or smaller volume of normal tissue result in fewer treatment complications, protons and charged particles provide the opportunity to improve the therapeutic ratio by increasing the tumor cure probability while simultaneously reducing the risk to normal tissue complications.*

The therapeutic ratio compares the healing aspects to the damaging possibilities. Needless to say, you want the most healing and the least damage.

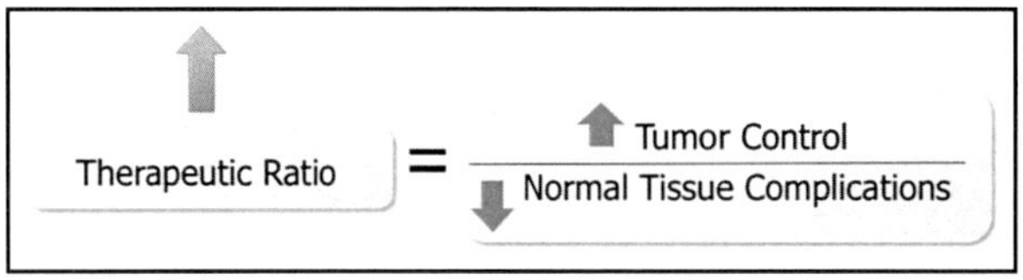

For the best result, these values should increase in the direction of the arrows. Proton therapy does exactly that.

I met on several occasions with Ben Robison, the Director of Medical Physics. He showed me on the computer how they created my personal dose plan, which filled twenty-two pages. One of the leading medical software companies in the world teamed up with Provision to inaugurate a very sophisticated software system for proton therapy, which Ben demonstrated for me. The following paragraphs come from Provision:

> *Provision Healthcare is partnering with leading treatment planning software developer, RaySearch Laboratories AB, to offer new user education at the Provision Center for Proton Therapy's state-of-the-art treatment and training facilities.*
>
> *Provision was the first proton therapy center to adopt the company's system, called RayStation, and has worked collaboratively*

with RaySearch since the launch of the Provision Center for Proton Therapy in January 2014.

"Over the past nearly two years, we have put RayStation through its paces, and we are pleased with the results. The physicists and medical dosimetrists who come for training will have a chance to learn from our clinical staff and see RayStation in action at a working medical center," said Niek Schreuder, chief medical physicist for Provision Center for Proton Therapy. "Our world-class proton therapy facility plus a modern, fully-equipped training center will provide both classroom and hands-on instruction for the staff who will be working with patients and physicians in treatment planning."

RaySearch markets the RayStation® treatment planning system to clinics all over the world. In addition, RaySearch's products are distributed through licensing agreements with leading medical technology companies. Their solutions are used successfully in over 2,500 clinics in more than 65 countries. RaySearch was founded in 2000 as a spin-off from Karolinska Institute in Stockholm, Sweden. The product development and research teams remain based at the head office in Stockholm, together with senior management and the central sales, marketing, and service organization. In less than fifteen years, the company has established a world-leading position in the field of advanced software for radiation therapy. Hundreds of thousands of cancer treatments delivered each year utilize RaySearch's algorithms and software products.

I saw the software in action as Ben put it through its paces. He started with the fused CT and MRI scan and physically drew color-coded perimeters around the prostate and other relevant organs. He could then turn the drawing in any direction with the shapes moving accordingly. He would point out, "Now here's the prostate. . ." and then turn the drawing to a different viewpoint and say, "Here are the lymph nodes you started treating today." Able to view everything from any angle he showed how he reached some dose areas from one side and some from the other.

Ben illustrated how most of the bladder would be exposed with intensity modified X-rays, taking a major hit of radiation. "Lymph nodes are where proton therapy really shines," he said. He compared pencil beam scanning to the way an ink jet printer puts down many tiny dots, with some dots darker (stronger) than others.

The lymph nodes form a "U" shape, following the pelvic bones much farther than I would have imagined. PBS can treat both arms of the "U" without crossing through the middle (by treating from each side, then stopping). X-rays must go all the way across (and continue out the body), thus affecting the middle area of the "U" with a full dose (see illustration on the next page).

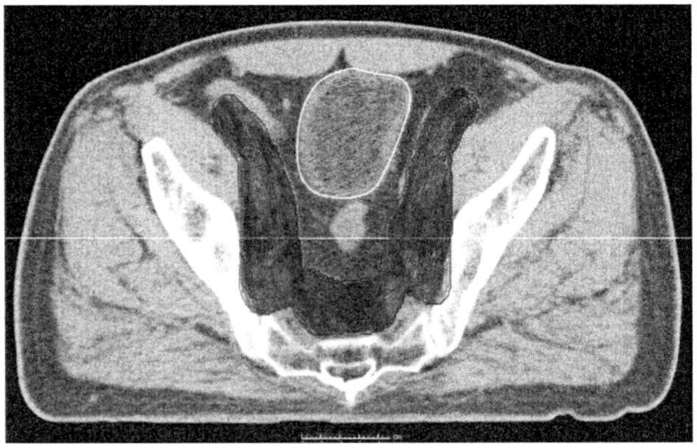

Above: The lymph nodes are colored in magenta, the bladder in yellow. The pelvic bones are white. PBS can treat the "U" shape from each side, whereas X-rays would go all the way across, massively affecting the bladder.

To cover the possibility of some variation, the dose covers a somewhat larger area than the target itself. The more precise the delivery, the less the size of the margin needs to be. The plan must also take into consideration possible movement by the patient. The standard margin is typically 3.5% at other proton centers, but a little less at Provision. In one direction, the margin should be within my SpaceOAR Hydrogel and thus spare any radiation to the rectum.

The bladder, however, touches the prostate; so the edge of it will be within the margin, which is the narrowest there. The lateral direction of the horizontal proton beams coming through the femur heads has the highest degree of uncertainty due to inherent discrepancies converting CT images from my simulation to proton algorithms. Margins, then, directly reflect uncertainty. If we were absolutely sure of all the factors and measurements, the margins would be infinitesimal.

Fortunately, there are no sensitive organs at risk in the horizontal direction so margins can be a little greater (say six or seven millimeters rather than three or four). For me personally, the dosimetrists graph every layer and every dot on an image of my anatomy as determined by the scans taken during my simulation. Hence the dose plan covered more than twenty pages.

These calculations give them the Planning Target Volume. They also consider the Clinical Target Volume, the actual cancerous areas that must be treated. A graph fuses the targets together. If they don't match, back to the drawing table. Done before treatment can begin, this process is called *robust optimization*, and also *inverse planning of margins*. In cases where circumstances change, a completely new dosimetry plan must be recalculated. "Robust" indeed.

During my proton therapy, on-going quality assurance verified the suitability of my plan. Quality assurance (QA) called for periodic CT scans to check the location of my gel and fiducial markers. They also looked at my daily X-rays. If you remember, for each treatment they took X-rays that showed my fiducial markers. These markers must line up within a certain range, indicated on the screen by lined areas called *grapes* *(see page 43)*. Every day my doctor examined these alignment images. He also approved any changes in my plan, such as the day they began treating the lymph nodes.

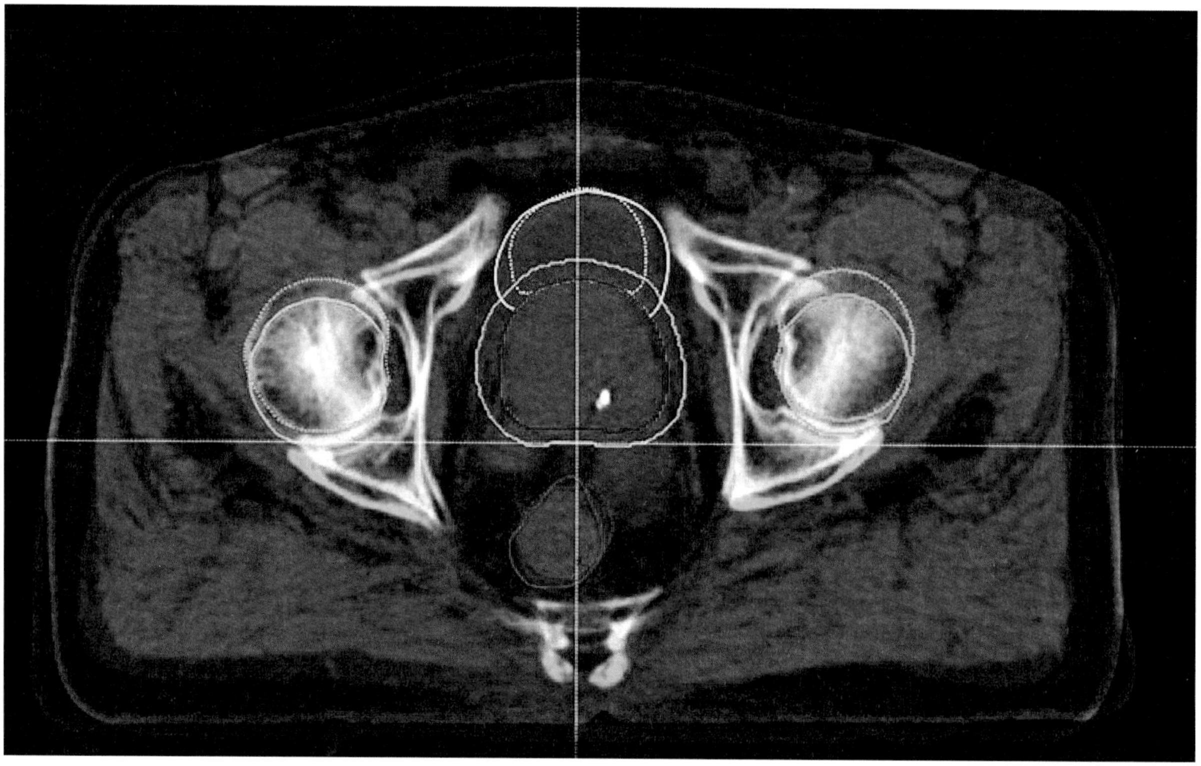

This fused picture of two CT scans from different days shows movement in most of the organs (bladder in yellow, femur heads left and right, rectum on the bottom) but none in the prostate itself (red). That's what really counts; so they verify the accuracy each day using the X-rays of my fiducial markers. The rest of the anatomy can vary slightly without affecting the treatment of the prostate.

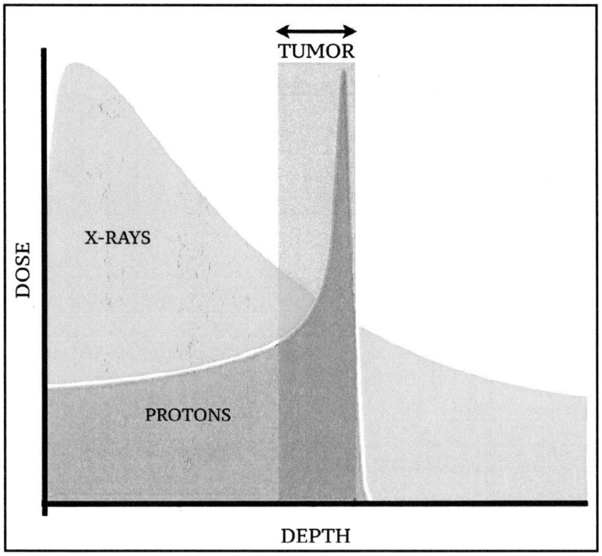

This iconic graph shows energy release. The orange represents protons, which at the end of their journey have a big spike in energy called the Bragg's Peak and then stop, with no exit dose. The blue area represents traditional single-beam X-rays which have a considerable entry dose and continue past the target (exit dose). This very popular graphic shows an important relationship, but doesn't reflect the fact that single beam X-rays are rarely used any more.

Notice how much less proton therapy affects the entry area. To avoid a large entry dose, X-rays with less energy are directed from different angles overlapping the tumor so the sum of the X-rays equals the desired total dose to the target while healthy tissue receives a reduced dose. The gray area on the graph, then, would have a lower slope. Nor are protons represented literally. Rather than a single Bragg's Peak, as shown, a group of Bragg's Peaks combine to form the spread-out Bragg's Peak (SOBP), as shown in the next illustration.

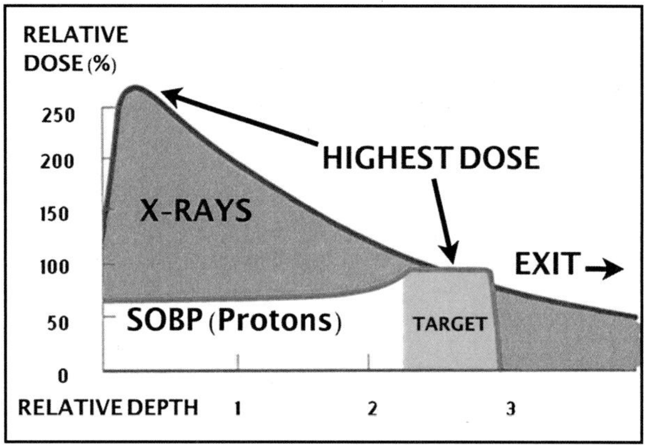

This shows the SOBP.

One clever article asked which you would rather have, a smart bomb (protons) or carpet bombing (X-rays).

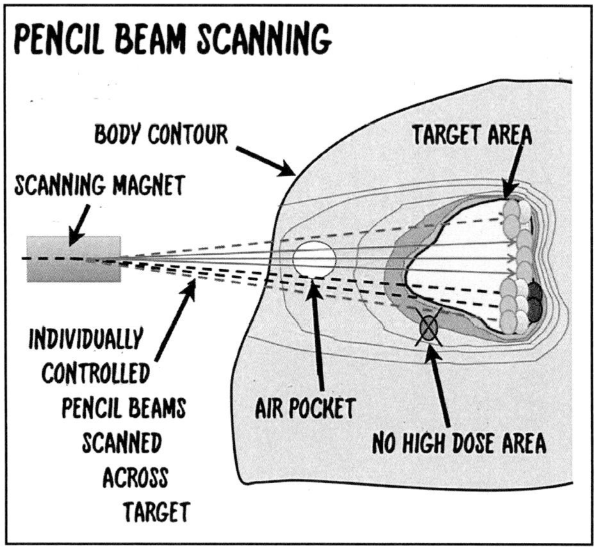

Pencil beam scanning doesn't cover wide areas like a blanket. Instead, it follows a designated pattern according to the dosimetry plan. The treated areas do not have to be contiguous. The spots can be accurately pinpointed to the designated targets even if intermittent.

To my email requesting the specific measurements for my treatment area(s), Ben responded thus.

> *For your Prostate Phase the distal range is 23.8cm with modulation width of 9.75 cm, thus the proximal end is 14 cm deep. For the nodal the range is 26.3 cm with a modulation width of 19.6 cm, thus a proximal end is 6.7 cm deep. For the Nodal field you have 31 layers and the prostate had 16 layers.*

Got that? Here is a chart summarizing a dosimetry plan very similar to my own, which was also sixteen layers.

Layer	Energy	Relative weight
1	188.9	2.63%
2	185.4	8.05%
3	181.9	13.52%
4	178.5	17.49%
5	175.1	14.09%
6	171.7	8.16%
7	168.4	8.16%
8	165.1	6.03%
9	161.9	5.11%
10	158.16	4.39%
11	156.8	3.70%
12	155.3	3.08%
13	152.1	2.16%
14	149.2	1.64%
15	145.8	1.21%
16	142.7	0.58%

Here is a detailed chart for a similar treatment to mine.

I originally thought my dose was 78 Gy (Gray, a measurement for radiation) for each fraction. I would have been fried! It was 78 Gy total for all of my thirty-nine treatments (2 Gy each).

Besides the dose strength, we can count the spots. I received sixteen layers from each side, one side with 1,800 spots and the other with 1,962 spots. Then, the seminal vesicles and lymph nodes increased the plan to thirty-one layers from the right side (with 5,314 spots) and thirty-two layers from the left side (with

5,276 spots). The spots overlap almost completely, being spread apart by a very small 2.45 mm. For my prostate target diameter of 9.75 cm (97.5 mm), one row would contain forty overlapping spots. Adding up the rows and layers easily totals thousands of spots.

One source I read states that the spots are laid down at the rate of four hundred per second. For my 5,276 spots, that would take thirteen seconds beam time, perhaps half a minute total for both sides. The rest of the time involves changing position from one side to the other, getting lined up properly (X-rays, merging scans, etc.), and the time it takes the degrader to change the energy between layers.

How does this dosimetry compare to other proton therapy centers? Although I didn't go to Prague for my proton therapy, I stayed in touch with Brooke Palmer. In my darkest days of research she was a guiding light, helping me to see the benefits of proton therapy. I wrote to Brooke about this book and asked some questions about their treatments, to see if they use a smaller number of treatments (called fractions).

She replied that they have three different treatment modalities, each with different dosimetry. Early stage and low risk cases call for five fractions, one administered every other day at 7.25 Gy per fraction (more than three times the energy of my fractions). The in between day gives a little more time for healthy tissue to recover. I haven't read about anyone in the United States offering as few as five fractions, or such a high dose, although a number of hypofractionated trials are being conducted.

The second modality at the proton therapy center in Prague prescribes nineteen fractions, for people who previously had surgery. Apparently they have quite a few such cases. The third modality, most closely resembling mine, uses twenty-one fractions at 3 Gy per fraction. They have settled on this proportion of fractions to doses, with twenty-one fractions = 63 Gy vs. my thirty-nine fractions = 78 Gy. The intent remains the same, to kill the cancer and spare the healthy tissue.

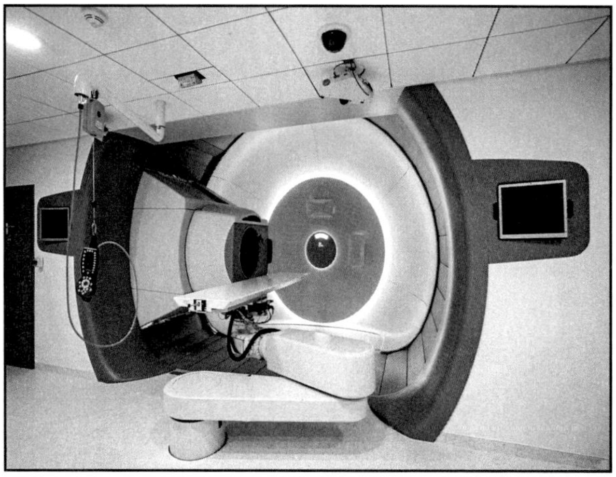

This is one of the gantries at the proton therapy center in Prague. See the list of centers at the end of the book for contact information.

The center in Prague benefits from the fact that medical insurance in England covers going there for treatments not locally available. Brexit (Britain's departure from the European Union) may have some effect on that policy. In addition, six proton therapy centers are in the planning stage for Britain and one has already opened.

As this chapter shows, much is taken into consideration to arrive at the correct dose and targeting. More recent versions of PBS have narrower beams and spots, which can zero in even more precisely on tumors. The IBA beam at Provision measured around 7 mm with a Bragg's Peak of around 15 mm. Smaller is not necessarily better in my case, as larger spots can be more efficient. If we were treating my brain, however, a spot of only a few millimeters might make a major difference.

Two additional treatment rooms at Provision opened in February of 2018. They have ProNova equipment with the latest PBS which will have an adjustable spot size. They are the only proton therapy center with two cyclotrons.

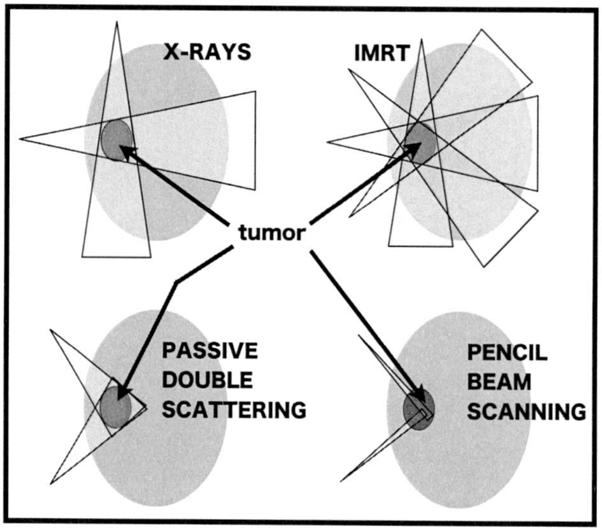

Here is a summary of the four types of radiation with which we should now be familiar, if not conversant.

CHAPTER 12 DIET AND LIFESTYLE

Linda and I continually read books and watch videos about proper diet and lifestyle. Our choices set us far apart from the Standard American Diet (SAD) to an extent that many would consider extreme. Even before we arrived in Knoxville, we adjusted our diet to our anticipated circumstances.

A sheet from Provision sent to us in Texas warned us to avoid certain foods to limit intestinal flatulence (gas). It included such things to eliminate as chewing gum, smoking, and sipping through a straw.

I'm told that flatulence is not a frivolous concern, as gas in the rectum can affect the position of the prostate, which in turn would throw off the accuracy of the treatment. On the X-ray used for positioning, the techs see gas as a big gray area. The patient may be asked to go to the bathroom to pass as much as possible. Otherwise, the red robin may be called into action. "What's a red robin?" I asked Cortney, one of the techs. She replied, "Not a hamburger," referring to the restaurant chain of the same name. Nor a bird. It's a kind of catheter used to release gas trapped in the rectum. I never thought I would be writing about such topics. Fortunately, I never had to use it.

Foods that produce gas
LEGUMES **Beans, baked beans, dry beans and peas, soy, lima**
DAIRY **Milk, ice cream, cheese, rich cream sauces**
VEGETABLES **Cruciferous vegetables, onions, cucumbers, asparagus**
FRUIT **Prunes, dried fruit, apricots**
HIGH-FAT FOODS **Deep fried anything, fried foods, fatty meats (ribs)**
LIQUIDS **Carbonated drinks of all kinds, beer,**
CAFFEINE **Coffee, tea** **Energy drinks** **Chocolate**

In addition to not eating the items listed here, the recommendations from Provision include using a stool softener (Docusate Sodium) and taking Beano throughout treatment. To my relief, they don't require an enema before each of my daily treatments as they do at some other proton centers.

I regret excluding some of my favorite foods. I live on broccoli, eating it almost every day. At home, I even put frozen broccoli in my smoothies (you can't taste it). And yes, most of the time, I do have a little gas. Now I had to change my diet to avoid it.

I found taking Beano with every meal made me constipated, hence the stool softener. Obsessive as usual, I did more research, accumulating nineteen pages of information from the internet about flatulence. This diligence on my part reflected my desire to fully comply with my treatment parameters. I established a diet and routine that served me very well. Here were the principles I followed.

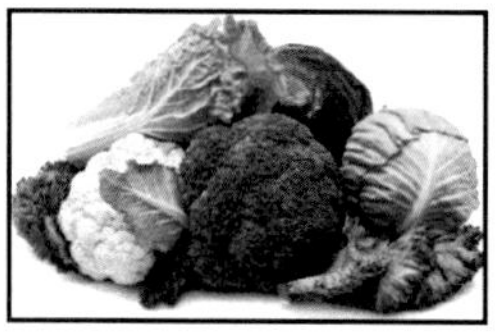

1. Avoid the items known to cause gas (see list).

2. You can have a meal three hours before treatment. In other words, breakfast. Keep it simple.

3. Make your own list. Keep a food journal if necessary to record what responses you have to particular foods.

4. Do what it takes to assure good digestion. Flatulence happens from incomplete digestion. I took supplements, including a probiotic and digestive enzymes. I also had some whole milk yogurt or Greek yogurt for the acidophilus and bifida. Yogurt decreases gas, as does buttermilk (which I hate). Avoid products full of sugar (which you should do anyway).

5. Reduce carbs, which cause intestinal bacteria to release hydrogen and methane. While the average person produces more than a liter of flatulence a day, the amount of gas goes way down on low carb diets. Fruit, I'm sorry to say, digests much like a carbohydrate, with the same resulting gas. Gluten can also be a gas producer. I happen to be gluten free so I rarely eat any wheat, spelt, kamut, farro, durum, bulgar or semolina. Oats have me puzzled, whether or not they have gluten.

6. Pay attention to *how* you eat, not just what you eat. Don't drink a lot of water with a meal, as it dilutes stomach acid and leads to incomplete digestion. If you want to strengthen your digestion, take a tablespoon of organic apple cider vinegar in a glass of warm water twenty minutes before a meal. Chew food well (thirty times, says Linda), especially carbs, as the mouth is the first stage of digestion. Chew with your mouth closed and don't talk while chewing as this makes you swallow air. Avoid straws. Relax. Stress and anxiety can make us breathe faster and thus take in more air.

7. Help your digestion. At Indian restaurants I always take some of the anise seeds to aid digestion. Peppermint does the same thing, as does ginger. Papaya is a rich source of valuable proteolytic enzymes that can greatly aid in the digestion of meat or other concentrated forms of protein.

8. Use Beano and Ducosate Sodium (stool softener) as needed. Beano and GasX do different things. Beano prevents the formation of gas whereas GasX works to reduce gas already there. Provision didn't say anything about GasX and I never tried it. Fiber greatly aids digestion, so every day I put some Benefiber in my drinking water. It dissolves

quickly and has no taste. You can also put it into juice or smoothies. (Benefiber is made of wheat dextrin, yet says it's gluten free.)

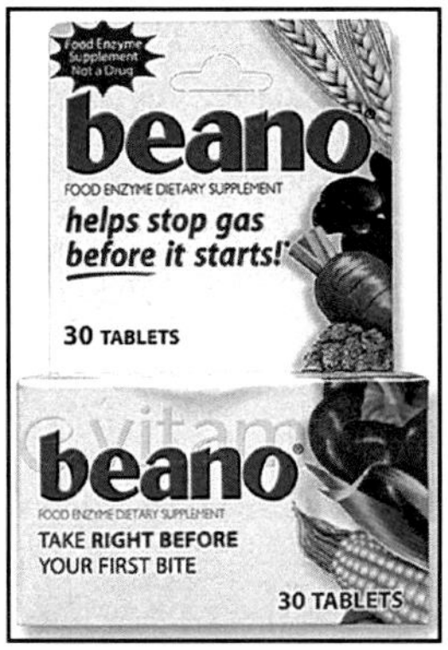

9. Avoid laxatives and artificial sweeteners. Laxatives excessively hurry the elimination process, creating gas in the process. Sugar alcohols and artificial sweeteners cause difficulties with digestion resulting in flatulence.

10. Ignore most advice about food combining. I remember decades ago reading *Diet for a Small Planet* (published in 1971) by Frances Moore Lappé and following her advice. Ten years later she wrote a book countering her advice, saying she got it wrong the first time.

The internet is rife with advice from so-called experts about food combining, but in the end (no pun intended) it's bunk. They suggest that different foods take different amounts of time to digest. If you eat a slow digester first (say, shell food) followed by a fast digester (say, fruit) then there will be problems. Many books and diets rely on this fallacy. Actually, your stomach mixes everything up together (they don't wait in line to be digested in the order swallowed) into a mixture called *chyme*. When the contents of your stomach pass to the small intestine, your pancreas goes into action and produces the right combination of enzymes (and bicarbonate to adjust the pH level to be more alkaline) resulting in proper digestion. The exception to food combining nonsense is Ayurveda, an ancient system for combining foods according to many criteria, not just digestion. Whew! I spent three days working on just this one point.

11. Avoid overeating. A huge meal can be hard to digest and lead to gas. It's much healthier to eat small meals with healthy snacks in between (fruit, celery, nuts).

12. Medicines, drugs, and some food additives can cause gas. These are good guidelines for general intestinal health, not just avoiding gas.

LIVE IT, DON'T DIET

Twice a week, Casey Coffey gave dietary presentations at Provision. I have been outraged many times in the past by dietitians who served as apologists for the food industry, who followed the flawed FDA food pyramid, or who promoted some bizarre theory. Casey, besides having great experience and credentials, lives what she teaches and makes good sense. Rather than summarizing my personal regime, I will restrict myself here to outlining what Casey teaches as the "official" dietary advice.

Her primary message can be summarized in one word: *balance*. To demonstrate this, she takes a plate and divides it in half, and then one side in half again, forming two quarters. The half is for vegetables, one quarter is for protein, and one quarter is for carbohydrates and fruit. For thirty years I followed a fairly strict vegetarian regime. As I get older, my doctors tell me I need more protein, to which I respond by putting protein powder in my smoothies.

Casey makes a strong point for protein at every meal and, of course, to avoid refined foods and too many carbs. That includes too much fruit, which is a shocker for me. I love fruit. So for those two months I strove to have protein with every meal and sometimes, no carbs (which are optional and can be completely avoided).

Typically in our refrigerator we had a jar of herring, some smoked salmon, prosciutto ham, and turkey bacon. For my new favorite lunch I fixed a sandwich made of two slices of turkey bacon, several leaves of lettuce and a fat tomato slice on tiny pieces of gluten-free bread (with the makings hanging out every side). This lunchtime delicacy had veggies, protein, and minimal carbs. I was full of energy and had no fatigue (a common side effect of X-rays). I decided to pay more attention to protein. Alas, when I got back home my cholesterol was high, especially the bad LDL part, so I went back to mostly a plant-based diet.

Meanwhile, at the top of Casey's plate is a small place for healthy oils and nuts. I've never had much regard for safflower oil or peanuts, but she seems to like them. All meals start with protein, to which you add plenty of vegetables and, if you must, some carbs. I made this chart of Casey's system.

You can download this chart from our website (see http://www.protontherapybook.com/cleanplatefull.pdf).

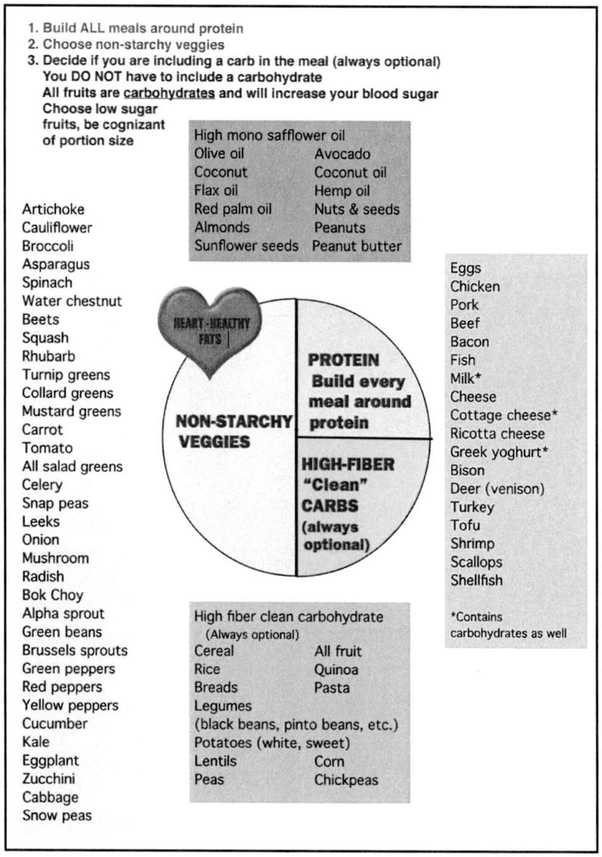

We met patients at Provision who, because of staying in hotels, went out to eat every meal. That made it very hard to maintain good eating habits.

Over the years I have followed many different diets, including macrobiotic, vegan, raw food, blood type, juicing, fasting, low fat, Paleo, South Beach, and vegetarian. In recent years, the Mediterranean Diet seems to have the most credibility. About a year ago, I read that low-fat diets have been misguided and actually led to our obesity epidemic. The body needs fat for taste and for nutrition. Low fat items, as with gluten free products, are likely to be loaded with too much salt and sugar.

Books by Dr. Mark Hyman convinced me that some kinds of fat are beneficial. But not just any fat. Basically all plant-based oils have far too much omega-6, which leads to inflammation and rejection by the body. I stay with virgin olive oil, avocado oil, or coconut oil. Virtually all restaurants fry things in genetically modified soybean oil or peanut oil or vegetable oil blends, which I avoid. We shouldn't be eating friend things anyway.

When I go to Whole Foods I don't find acceptable many of the presumably healthy products, especially chips fried in heavily omega-6 oils. Then at Trader Joe's, I find they load many of their branded items with sugar or other sweeteners, whether organic or not. And those are health food stores. Regular grocery stores are worse, where I won't touch about 90% of the items. It's no wonder we have a health crisis in this country. We have really gone astray when it comes to healthy eating.

Many people don't welcome changing their eating habits. "I would rather die than give up my pasta." That's a high price to pay. Maybe giving up poor quality foods seems like a sacrifice, but in the end, good health is its own reward. My current challenge involves giving up sugar, which is in just about everything.

Very often you hear that you should have five servings a day of fruit or vegetables, as if they are equivalent. If you look again at the divided plate, fruit is placed with the carbohydrates, not with the vegetables. So it matters whether you choose fruit or vegetables. You can have all the vegetables you want, whereas carbs and fruit should be limited. I had never considered this distinction before hearing Casey. So, of course, I went to the internet and found some information on www.livestrong.com, as follows.

Carbs are a macronutrient that can be divided into three distinct components called starches, sugars and fibers. The structure of carbs found in fruits and in grains differs slightly, but both kinds of carbs when digested contribute to raising your blood sugar levels after a meal. Only fiber does not raise blood sugar, because your body does not digest or absorb fiber. You can get fiber in fresh fruits but not fruit juices, as well as in whole grains but not in refined grains; fiber promotes regular and easy bowel movements.

The main type of carbs found in fruits is sugar, including varying proportions of fructose, glucose and sucrose. Fructose and glucose consist of one single molecule of sugar, while sucrose is two molecules of sugar bonded together. These sugars can quickly be digested and absorbed into your bloodstream.

The carbs found in grains are mainly in the form of starches. Starch is a long chain made of many molecules of glucose attached to one another. After eating grains, the enzyme amylase can easily break down starches to obtain single molecules of glucose, which can be absorbed from your intestines into your bloodstream.

The carbs in fruits are sometimes called simple carbs, and the carbs in grains are sometimes called complex carbs. However, the Harvard School of Public Health says that this classification is not helpful in assessing the healthfulness of different carbs; it says the glycemic index is more appropriate to distinguish between carbs that can make your blood sugar levels peak and those that help keep them more stable.

Whole fruits have a low glycemic index, which is beneficial for controlling your blood sugar levels. The glycemic index of grains varies depending on many factors. White bread, pretzels, bagels, white rice and most breakfast cereals, even the unsweetened brands, have high glycemic index values and can make your blood sugar levels spike. On the other hand, quinoa, millet, pasta, sourdough bread, steel-cut oats and basmati rice have lower values and can help prevent large variations in your blood sugar levels after eating.

People facing diabetes, or who are pre-diabetic, should especially keep an eye on the glycemic index of foods. The statement above that whole fruits have a low glycemic index is music to my ears, but I don't think it takes into account the different values for different fruits.

You can go to the internet and get charts that show the glycemic index of various foods. With regard to fruits, here are some values I found. Try to stay under a rating of fifty. Some of my favorite fruits rate much higher than that. I still eat them, but in smaller portions.

Grapefruit	25
Apricots (dried)	31
Apples	38
Pears	38
Plums	39
Peaches	42
Oranges	44
Grapes	46
Kiwi fruit	53
Bananas	54
Fruit cocktail	55
Mangoes	56
Apricots (fresh)	57
Raisins	64
Pineapple	66
Dates	103

Some health experts extol the virtues of dates, finding them full of minerals and vitamins. They call them "nature's candy." Yet consider their stratospheric glycemic rating. This kind of conflicting advice drives me crazy. I put three dates into the homemade almond milk that I make in my VitaMix (one quart). That gives it just enough sweetness.

One study found that twenty servings of fresh fruit per day was *beneficial* and did not affect overall blood sugar levels. It gave the green light to eat unlimited amounts of fruit of all kinds.

I wish a very simple health index could indicate the relative benefits of one food over another. But who would write it? Corporate interests fund junk science that they promote as authentic, like Coca-Cola saying sugar isn't bad, you just need to count calories. The FDA had to stop Twinkies from advertising that they were a wholesome snack for our children.

If I pick up a product and see the ingredients take an inch of fine print, I don't even read it. I just put it back on the shelf. Walk into any grocery store and you will find a vast area around the bakery with shelf after shelf filled with white flour, sugar, highly refined carbs, high fructose corn syrup and empty calories in the form of white bread, donuts, cookies, cakes, and other items. They're poison. Yet they must serve a big demand given the size of the display. The health food section is at the end of a shelf in some obscure aisle.

Where to start? Use Casey's clean plate system, reject highly refined and junk foods, reject fried foods and sodas, and buy organic even if it costs more. Start somewhere, take one step at a time, and arrive at a healthier lifestyle that will allow you greater quality of life, happiness, and longevity.

In Knoxville, we went to a local vegetarian/vegan/healthy restaurant called Tomatohead. In a weak moment, I asked for fries with my veggie burger. "We don't have fries," the server responded. Then the shocker. "We don't even have a fryer in the kitchen." You go, girl.

Avoid artificial sweeteners, artificial food dyes, energy drinks and highly processed food of any kind, high fructose corn syrup, MSG, potassium bromate, sodium nitrite and sodium nitrate. If people refuse to buy these products, manufacturers would quit making them. (Food shouldn't be manufactured, anyway.) Good luck.

Cancer is a wakeup call to refine our diet in the direction of better health. It has been shown that cancer thrives on sugar. One anti-cancer diet is to eliminate all sweets. For me, I shoot for eliminating 80%, allowing the odd dessert here and there.

CHAPTER 13 INNER HEALING

A number of books consider surviving cancer to be a miracle reflecting direct divine intervention. Although I may not take quite that position, I do believe that our lives in general and healing in particular reflect spiritual principles that reflect the quality of our inner lives.

We've all heard from people who say getting cancer was the best thing that ever happened to them because it improved the quality of their lives. Franciscan monk Richard Rohr predicts that we are likely to just slide along through life until some traumatic event, some sudden impetus, forces us into a deeper spiritual awareness. I always felt he was exaggerating, but I represent that exact pattern, wanting to meditate more and go deeper but somehow never getting around to it.

Then my prostate cancer showed up, spurring a time of transformation. It gave me the kick in the pants that I needed. After all, I was diagnosed at age seventy-two. How much longer did I expect to wait? Even though Linda and I teach about the benefits of spiritual aging, I was being half-hearted about it. Not any more.

In Knoxville, I went to see Jean Wilhoite, a holistic nurse and Healing Touch practitioner. She addressed my mission of healing in terms of energy and balance and metaphysical considerations. *Meta* means "beyond," hence metaphysical means beyond the physical. Here are some passages from my journal.

During my ninety-minute Healing Touch session, in which she reordered and balanced the energy surrounding me, sometimes lightly touching me, sometimes moving her hands just above my body, I had a number of important realizations (revelations).

The first was about deserving. That was a big one. There's some part of me that doesn't feel deserving of being healed. I have read that all illness is lack of forgiveness. In this case, it's apparently myself I'm not forgiving. By not feeling deserving of healing, I block the way for it to happen. I call that a constriction. Well, that's exactly the problem, isn't it. I'm too constricted to pee.

Secondly, I thought about flow. I realized that, too, is the physical manifestation I have created. My urine won't flow. Spiritually, I need to get out of the way. I need to turn off the ego. One might say that I need to empty myself. Oh my, another metaphor. I need to empty my bladder.

This is completely in accord with my understanding that the physical world is just the effect; cause lies in the invisible world, our inner world. That's not where traditional medicine goes, nor is it interested in doing so. It deals with symptoms and appearances.

All of this makes me think of the time I spend on the table receiving proton therapy. I want to visualize the protons entering my prostate and obliterating the cancer cells. I want to welcome them as a part of my healing. But once on the table, I tend to be distracted. I try to concentrate on the protons, but soon my mind wanders. Why am I almost incapable of seeing the protons as healing agents?

I seem unwilling to be healed. I'm not in rapport with the flow of the protons. All of this reflects my emotional and spiritual issues. If I can make progress in these, it will enhance my healing.

For several days the theme of "flow" kept showing up in various places, such as this poem from John O'Donohue:

> *I would love to live*
> *Like a river flows,*
> *Carried by the surprise*
> *Of its own unfolding.*

I discovered that the divine Flow isn't personal. I'm not required to be perfect or right, belong to a certain group, or even understand Flow. Jesus has no list of pre-qualifications. He doesn't check if the people he heals are Jewish, gay, baptized, or in their first marriage. He asks only one question, in various ways: "Do you want to be healed?"

Linda took a walk along the water course at Dowell Springs only to find it dry. The recirculating pump was turned off while they performed some kind of maintenance. So there was no flow. The ponds sat empty, full of leaves and debris. What a great opportunity to clean them out and make everything fully functional.

Others who have written about proton therapy have included references to more traditional religious beliefs. In *Calming the Storm: A Christ-Follower's Victory Over Cancer*, Don Denton attributes everything good in his cancer experience to God and every delay or stumbling block to the devil. I personally don't lean toward such a literal black-and-white perspective. Sometimes problems turn out to be a great blessing. We often can't judge what's best for ourselves or others.

John Piper, in his booklet "Don't Waste Your Cancer," makes a good point. Rather than being angry or depressed or fearful, prostate cancer can lead to important spiritual growth. His preface starts like this.

> *I originally wrote this on the eve of prostate-cancer surgery. I believed then, and I believe now, in God's power to heal—by miracle and by medicine. I believe it is right and good to pray for both kinds of healing. Cancer is not wasted when it is healed by God. He gets the glory, and that is why cancer*

exists. So not to pray for healing may waste our cancer.

(We waste our cancer if we. . .)

. . . don't hear in our own groanings the hope-filled labor pains of a fallen world.
. . . do not believe it is designed for us by God.
. . . believe it is a curse and not a gift.
. . . seek comfort from the odds rather than from God.
. . . refuse to think about death.
. . . think that "beating" cancer means staying alive rather than cherishing Christ.
. . . spend too much time reading about cancer and not reading about God.
. . . let it drive us into solitude instead of deepen our relationships with manifest affection.
. . . grieve as those who have no hope.
. . . treat sin as casually as before.
. . . fail to use it as a means of witness to the truth and glory of Christ.

Were I to make my own list, it would be quite different. For example, I don't think God conspires to give anyone cancer just to be glorified. Glorifying God, however, can be extremely healing. I agree with Piper, we can all gain by not wasting our cancer but instead using it to deepen our connection to Something greater than ourselves, however each of us chooses to define that force.

Miracles have abounded in my prostate journey. They say you will find no atheists in foxholes. Nor in cancer wards I would add. Given how long my PSA numbers had been high, the cancer could have spread, which would have led to some kind of systemic treatment that I would have found totally unacceptable. Instead, I have been the recipient of miracles. I want to embrace my cancer experience, not waste it.

Did I bring prostate cancer on myself? Oh yes, along with everything else in my life. I don't believe any of us are victims. Everything has a purpose. We write our own scripts, whether consciously or otherwise. Taking responsibility, I've spent many hours of reflection, meditation, and prayer. When walking to the fitness center near our home in San Antonio along a path through a lovely green area, I would sit on a bench along the way, talking out loud to myself and Whomever Else may be listening. I repeated my affirmation, "Happy, Healthy and Whole."

I don't believe the Universe hears the word "No." If I say, "I *don't* want to get cancer" the universe hears "I *want* to get cancer." The more I dwell on what I don't want to happen, the more it comes to pass. Saying I don't want cancer gives energy to it. Suppose you want help from higher sources and you say "I don't want to go to California." How can they help you? Where *do* you want to go? You have to say, "I want to go to Wisconsin," or whatever. Affirmations should never contain a negative or they become negations. Therefore, I repeated phrases like "I am cancer free" or "the cancer is gone." Mostly, I preferred just to say that I'm happy, healthy, and whole, sometimes also adding "healed." This reflected what I want to manifest.

Did my actions and affirmations made any difference? In August, prior to going to Provision, I had another PSA test. My number went down ten percent from 16.0 in May to 14.4. I suppose it could have been a fluke or a statistical variation, but my actions may also have caused the cancer to withdraw and not metastasize. I considered that to be a spiritual breakthrough, which gave me great encouragement. I even considered delaying my treatment to see if my PSA would continue to decline, but decided against such a radical action.

I will never totally resolve all of my issues, of course. Spirituality is a lifelong (and life giving) process. Cancer puts everything on a front burner, raising priorities and demanding attention. I haven't wasted my cancer.

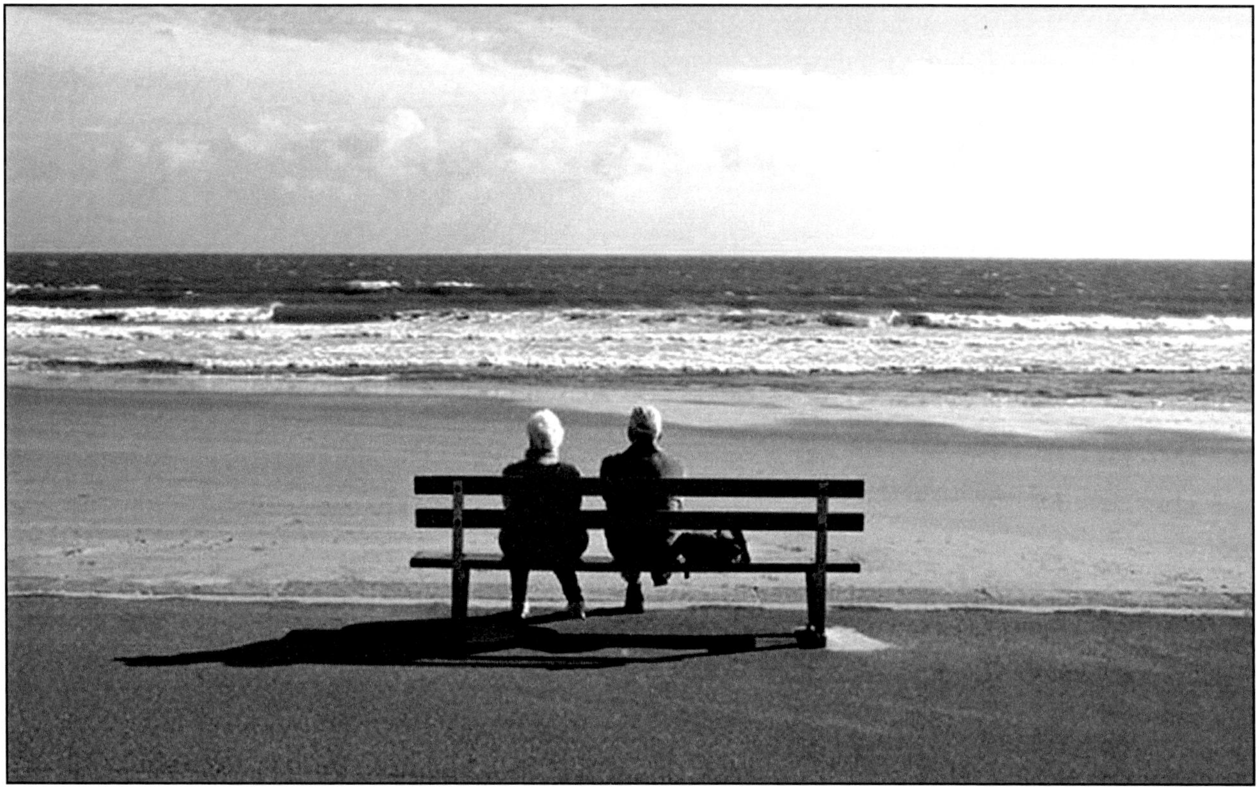

CHAPTER 14 MORE ABOUT MEDICARE

The prospect of Medicare coverage saved me from surgery and made proton therapy possible. I'm not unique. The same can be true for anyone over sixty-five who wants to be treated with proton therapy for most cancers, and especially prostate. The key is to be included in a type of trial called a registry, which follows you for life, in return for which Medicare pays 80% of the allowable charges for proton therapy. I heard of one case in which a qualified person hadn't yet started his Medicare. He did so and then came to Provision for treatment by joining the registry.

Early on, I hesitated to get my hopes up. Still, going to Europe seemed financially impossible, even at half the cost I would pay out-of-pocket in the United States.

I insisted that Provision send me copies of the actual documents so I could confirm the details in black and white. Then, for this book, I went into much more depth to assure the accuracy of my advice. Following are relevant portions of vital Medicare documentation taken from their own website.

Local Coverage Determination (LCD):
Radiology: Proton Beam Therapy (L34282)

Links in PDF documents are not guaranteed to work. To follow a web link, please use the MCD Website.

Contractor Information

Contractor Name	Contract Number	Contract Type
Cahaba Government Benefit Administrators®, LLC	10301	MAC - Part A

Back to Top

LCD Information

Document Information

LCD ID
L34282

Original ICD-9 LCD ID
L33070

LCD Title
Radiology: Proton Beam Therapy

Jurisdiction
Tennessee

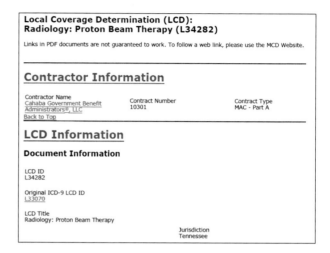

Because of the illegible type above, I reproduce the content below.

Local Coverage Determination (LCD)
Radiology: Proton Beam Therapy (L34282)
Links in PDF documents are not guaranteed to work. To follow a web link, please use the MCD Website.
Contractor Information
Contractor name:
Cahaba Government Benefit Administrators®, LLC
Contract number: 10301
Contract Type: MAC - Part A
LCD Information
LCD ID: L34282
Original ICD-9 LCD ID: L33070
LCD Title: Radiology: Proton Beam Therapy
Jurisdiction: Tennessee

Cahaba Government Benefit Administrators, LLC, an independent contractor called a MAC (Medicare Administrative Contractor) administers Alabama, Georgia, and Tennessee. Note the document above indicates *local* coverage determination (LCD), more specifically, for Tennessee, the one that pertains to Provision.

Medicare depends on MACs to do much of its regional business. Coverage can differ from one geographical area to another. L34282 represents the number that Medicare assigns the document that determines coverage, which does not pertain to any other region other than the one covered by Cahaba. This document gives more details.

LCD - Local Coverage Determination (LCD) for Radiology: Proton Beam Therapy (L33070) (This was the previous registration number, now L34282)
Posted March 12, 2014 in Part A/B (Updated)
The 'Indications' section for Group 2 and Documentation Requirement #2 were updated to include the use of modifier Q0 (zero) when billing for Group 2 Indication. Group 2 indications define conditions that are still under investigation and may be covered when the LCD criteria are met. There is no change in the effective date or coverage.

LCDs are located on the Medicare Coverage Database (MCD), which can be accessed from the 'Local Coverage Determination (LCD) & Articles' page of the 'Medical Review' sections on the Cahaba GBA website (select 'LCDs' for your state). Providers are encouraged to review this LCD to ensure compliance.

So far we see that private contractors administer Medicare on a regional level, in this case by Cahaba. The second document shows how Group 2 coverage meets the criteria of the LCDs, the local coverage determination. Group 1 comprises a list of conditions which Medicare covers outright. Group 2 contains a list of additional conditions covered only if they meet certain criteria.

Group 2

This section defines conditions that are still under investigation and may be covered when the patient is:

- enrolled in an IRB-approved clinical trial which meets the 'standards of scientific integrity and relevance to the Medicare population' described in the CMS Internet Only Manual (IOM): Medicare National Coverage Determinations (NCD) Manual (Pub 100-03), Chapter 1, Section 20.32 B.3.a-k;

or

- enrolled in a national or regional clinical registry compliant with the principles established in AHRQ's 'Registries for Evaluating Patient Outcomes: A User's Guide', such as the Registry for Prostate Cancer Radiosurgery (RPCR).

The second bullet directly applies to Provision's registry. Hence, coverage for 80% of allowable expenditures.

The next document outlines the medical conditions covered under LCD clinical trial regulations.

1. Unresectable lung cancers and upper abdominal/ peri-diaphragmatic cancers.
2. Advanced stage, unresectable pelvic tumors including those with peri-aortic nodes or malignant lesions of the cervix.
3. Unresectable breast tumors in proximity to the heart.
4. Unresectable pancreatic and adrenal tumors.
5. Skin cancer with microscopic perineural/cranial nerve invasion of the skull base.
6. Unresectable malignant lesions of the liver, biliary tract, anal canal and rectum.
7. Prostate cancer, non-metastatic.

Unresectable refers to a malignancy which can't be surgically removed, due either to the number of metastatic foci or because of location in a surgical danger zone. Of course, number seven pertains to this discussion, prostate cancer.

The registry at Provision covers proton therapy generally, not specific cancer types, hence the list. There you have, in black and white, the three elements that must all fall into place: the LCD, the registry, and a condition qualifying for the registry.

No other center I contacted mentioned having a registry, local coverage, or even Medicare in general. When I called proton therapy centers and mentioned that I have United Healthcare insurance, they replied apologetically that in their experience, my insurance would not cover proton therapy. Period. End of conversation.

People ask why I went to Knoxville and not one of the two centers in Texas, one of them being the famous M. D. Anderson. Very simple. The other centers never mentioned Medicare coverage to me (even if they might offer it, a grievous error on the part of the telephone receptionist). Provision has a clear connection to Medicare, and so I went there. Period.

In 2016, the Texas Center for Proton Therapy in Irving, Texas (near Dallas) was in the process of joining the Provision registry, which would lead to similar coverage by Medicare. More on that later. In my case, no one else offered any additional help except for Provision. It shows how good management and focus on essentials can bring business. Other centers could certainly learn a thing or two from Provision when it comes to caring for patients, as I discovered in my very first telephone call.

If you want to know about national registries, see scholarly articles on the subject at: http://www.effectivehealthcare.ahrq.gov. A list of trials can be found on the website www.clinicaltrials.gov. The Provision trial is number NCT02070328. I looked into trials before I found Provision, even writing to the Mayo Clinic about a trial they are doing comparing proton therapy and IMRT. However, by the time they responded (several weeks later) I was already at Provision.

I asked Provision for more details about medicare coverage and received the following:

Other states may apply to be on a local registry, it can also be used in conventional radiation in some cases. The goal of a registry is to track clinical outcomes. Medicare has considered protons for prostate as "Medically Necessary" since 1997. The cancer registry requirement is a regional requirement. Not all Medicare carriers require this. There is no "National Coverage Determination" or "NCD" for proton therapy, only "Local Coverage Determination" or "LCD". This simply means that the national "Centers for Medicare Services" or "CMS" has not established a set policy for proton therapy.

This implies that some regions may cover proton therapy for prostate cancer under other criteria. The map below shows MACs in the United States.

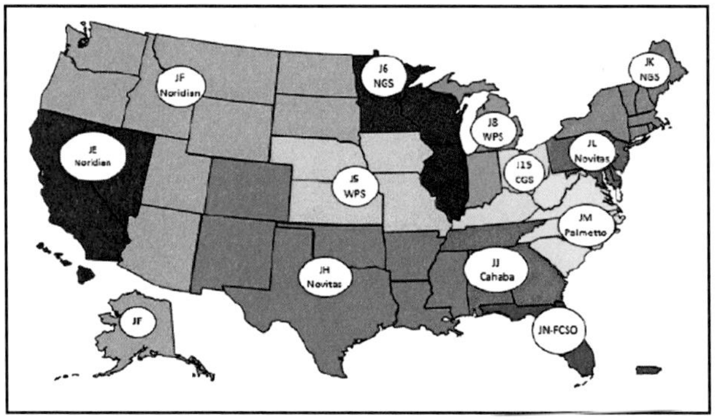

Alabama	Cahaba Government Benefit Administrators
Alaska	Noridian Healthcare Solutions LLC
American Samoa	"
Arizona	"
Arkansas	Novitas Solutions
California	Noridian Healthcare Solutions LLC
Colorado	Novitas Solutions
Connecticut	(None)
Delaware	Novitas Solutions
Washington D.C.	"
Florida	First Coast Service Options Inc.
Georgia	Cahaba Government Benefit Administrators
Guam	Noridian Healthcare Solutions LLC
Hawaii	"
Idaho	"
Illinois	(None)
Indiana	(None)
Iowa	(None)
Kansas	(None)
Kentucky	(None)
Louisiana	Novitas Solutions
Maine	(None)
Maryland	Novitas Solutions
Massachusetts	(None)
Michigan	(None)
Minnesota	(None)
Mississippi	Novitas Solutions
Missouri	(None)
Montana	Noridian Healthcare Solutions LLC
Nebraska	(None)
Nevada	Noridian Healthcare Solutions LLC

New Hampshire	(None)
New Jersey	Novitas Solutions
New Mexico	“
New York	(None)
North Carolina	(None)
North Dakota	Noridian Healthcare Solutions LLC
Ohio	(None)
Oklahoma	Novitas Solutions
Oregon	Noridian Healthcare Solutions LLC
Pennsylvania	Novitas Solutions
Puerto Rico	First Coast Service Options Inc.
Rhode Island	(None)
South Carolina	(None)
South Dakota	Noridian Healthcare Solutions LLC
Tennessee	Cahaba Government Benefit Administrators
Texas	Novitas Solutions
Utah	Noridian Healthcare Solutions LLC
Vermont	(None)
Virgin Islands	First Coast Service Options Inc.
Virginia	(None)
Washington	Noridian Healthcare Solutions LLC
West Virginia	(None)
Wisconsin	(None)
Wyoming	Noridian Healthcare Solutions LLC

I looked up the actual listing for Provision's trial, which is sponsored by The Center for Biomedical Research, LLC, a sister company to Provision in Knoxville. Note that Ackerman Cancer Center in Jacksonville, Florida, is also on this registry. That's not the big center at the University of Florida but rather, a private clinic with a single treatment room. For them to be included, I would think the Florida MAC, namely First Coast Service Options Inc., should list this trial but I can't find it. To understand this process I leaned on Brittany Price (Billing Specialist), Kristi Simcox (Research Coordinator), and Susan Owenby (Clinical Research) with many questions, which they

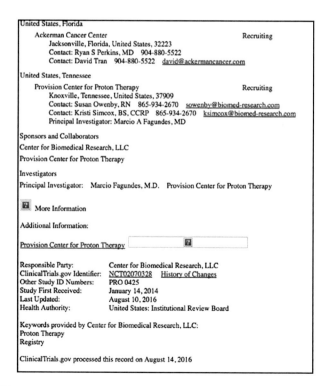

United States, Florida

Ackerman Cancer Center — Recruiting
Jacksonville, Florida, United States, 32223
Contact: Ryan S Perkins, MD 904-880-5522
Contact: David Tran 904-880-5522 david@ackermancancer.com

United States, Tennessee

Provision Center for Proton Therapy — Recruiting
Knoxville, Tennessee, United States, 37909
Contact: Susan Owenby, RN 865-934-2670 sowenby@biomed-research.com
Contact: Kristi Simcox, BS, CCRP 865-934-2670 ksimcox@biomed-research.com
Principal Investigator: Marcio A Fagundes, MD

Sponsors and Collaborators

Center for Biomedical Research, LLC

Provision Center for Proton Therapy

Investigators

Principal Investigator: Marcio Fagundes, M.D. Provision Center for Proton Therapy

More Information

Additional Information:

Provision Center for Proton Therapy

Responsible Party:	Center for Biomedical Research, LLC
ClinicalTrials.gov Identifier:	NCT02070328 History of Changes
Other Study ID Numbers:	PRO 0425
Study First Received:	January 14, 2014
Last Updated:	August 10, 2016
Health Authority:	United States: Institutional Review Board

Keywords provided by Center for Biomedical Research, LLC:
Proton Therapy
Registry

ClinicalTrials.gov processed this record on August 14, 2016

patiently answered again and again (as well as reading sections of my manuscript). Here's the full scoop on the registry.

Registry Study for Proton Therapy Clinical Outcomes and Long-Term Follow-up (Registry)
This study is currently recruiting participants. Verified August 2016 by Center for Biomedical Research, LLC
Sponsor: Center for Biomedical Research, LLC
Collaborator: Provision Center for Proton Therapy
Information provided by (Responsible Party): Center for Biomedical Research, LLC
ClinicalTrials.gov Identifier: NCT02070328
First received: January 14, 2014
Last updated: August 10, 2016
Last verified: August 2016

▶ ***Purpose***

Proton *therapy is a limited medical resource that is more expensive than conventional X-ray therapy. To correctly measure the success of* ***proton*** *therapy in treating different conditions, it is important to check a patient's health status after their treatment is finished. Checking on the progress of patients over many years (called long-term follow-up) is needed because the long-term effects of* ***proton*** *therapy are not well known.*
Study type: Observational (Patient Registry)
Study design: Observation Model: Case control.
Target Follow-Up Duration: 25 Years
Official Title: Registry Study for Proton Therapy Clinical Outcomes and Long-Term Follow-up
Further study details as provided by Center for Biomedical Research, LLC:

Primary Outcome Measures:
Long-term follow-up maintaining regular, lifetime contact with subjects in order to obtain current identification, contact information, and self/parent-reported health status in order to obtain a better understanding of overall treatment strategies and patient benefits of treatment.

Secondary Outcome Measures:
Performing retrospective research studies on diseases treated with proton therapy throughout the United States. Permitting review of medical record information contained within the Registry to identify subjects who may be eligible for participation in future research studies conducted at the Proton Therapy Institution where the participant was treated. Obtaining the permission of Research Registry participants to be contacted to ascertain their interest in participating in future research studies being conducted at their participating Proton Therapy Institution for which it appears (i.e., based on medical information contained within the Research Registry) they may be eligible.
Estimated Enrollment: 300
Study Start Date: December, 2013
Estimated Completion Date: January, 2022
Detailed Description: The objective of this research protocol is the development of a national Proton Therapy Center Registry for the purpose of:

Performing retrospective research studies on diseases treated with proton therapy throughout the United States.

Maintaining regular, lifetime contact with subjects in order to obtain current identification, contact information, and self/parent-reported health status in order to obtain a better understanding of overall treatment strategies and patient benefits of treatment.

Permitting review of medical record information contained within the Registry to identify subjects who may be eligible for participation in future research studies conducted at the Proton Therapy Institution where the participant was treated. Obtaining the permission of Research Registry participants to be contacted to ascertain their interest in participating in future research studies being conducted at their participating Proton Therapy Institution for which it appears (i.e., based on medical information contained within the Research Registry) they may be eligible.

▶ ***Eligibility***

Gender(s): Both
Accept Heathy Volunteers: No

Sampling Method: Non-probability Sample Study Population: Patients who are seen/treated at proton therapy centers
Inclusion Criteria: All subjects who are receiving or seeking medical care at the participating Proton Therapy Center will be invited to participate in the Research Registry.
Exclusion Criteria: Subjects who do not agree to participate
Please refer to this study by its ClinicalTrials.gov identifier: NCT02070328
Locations:
Ackerman Cancer Center
Jacksonville, Florida 32223
Contact: David Tran
Tel: 904-880-6622
Email: david@ackermancancer.com
Provision CARES Proton Therapy Center Knoxville
Knoxville, Tennessee 37909
Contact: Kristi Simcox
Tel: 865.934.2670
ksimcox@biomed-research.com
Principal Investigator (PI)
Original: Marcio A. Fagundes, MD
Currently: J. Ben Wilkinson MD

The number of participants and end date can change. As of November, 2016 there were 1,317 registrants of which 695 were for prostate cancer.

The registry originated at Indiana University in Bloomington, Indiana. When Indiana decommissioned their center, Provision became the lead sponsor. However, to be a registry requires more than one sponsor. Hence Ackerman Cancer Center and soon, the Texas Center for Proton Therapy.

Had the Texas center been already on the registry, and had I known about it, I would likely have gone there rather than Knoxville, as it's closer to my home in San Antonio.

If you are considering proton therapy and you are not old enough for Medicare coverage, I would suggest looking into possible trial participation paid for by the party doing the trial. Go to this website: www.clinicaltrials.gov.

The last time I checked it showed 277,864 studies from fifty states and 204 countries. Three trials caught my eye.
1. M. D Anderson, about quality of life with proton therapy (NCT00561444).
2. The University of Pennsylvania Abramson Cancer Center, requiring a PSA of less than 10 (NCT01045226).
3. Same sponsor as above, a study of the efficacy of yoga to counter side effects, but it includes both photons (X-rays) and protons.

The Medicare website confirms the concept of trials and registries as follows.

Clinical Research studies
How often is it covered?
Medicare covers clinical research studies which test different types of medical care, like how well a cancer drug works. These studies help doctors and researchers see if a new treatment works and is safe. Medicare Part A (Hospital Insurance) and/or Medicare Part B (Medical Insurance) cover some costs, like office visits and tests and in certain qualifying clinical research studies.

Who's eligible?
All people with Part A and Part B are covered in qualifying studies.

<u>Your Costs in Original Medicare</u>
You may have to pay 20% of the Medicare-approved amount depending on the treatment you get. The Part B deduction may apply.
Medicare will help pay for some of your costs if you join a covered clinical research study.

Read that last sentence again. It was music to my ears. The cost of such coverage to Medicare for this and thousands of other studies boggles the mind, running into billions of dollars. Medicare seriously supports research.

Millions of registrants are being tracked and studied, filling out evaluation forms, accumulating data. It would take a huge bureaucracy to keep track of all of this. Medicare found a solution. Since their payment helps support the research sponsor(s) and collaborator(s), why not put the burden of documentation on them? And so they do. Do they pay Provision anything for its registry? Here's what they told me.

There is no funding for conducting the registry trial coming to Provision Center for Proton Therapy. The staff it takes to conduct the study and collect the follow up data for the patient's life is costly to the center but necessary for our Medicare patients.

Suppose Provision's registry goes for twenty years, with six hundred registrants per year. That would total twelve thousand participants filling out reports every six months, plus thousands more from the Ackerman Center and Texas Center for Proton Therapy. With such an expense and long-term commitment, you can see why many centers don't care to get involved, finding it easier to join an existing study. How do they pay for the cost of conducting and managing the registry?

For one, they charge others who join the trial. Ackerman and Texas pay management fees. Beginning your own registry requires finding your way through a blizzard of red tape and requirements.

I wonder why Provision doesn't advertise nationally that if you have Medicare and a qualifying condition, you can get proton therapy. I think they would draw in many more people, a win-win for both parties.

How exactly does a proton therapy center join an existing registry? Susan Owenby described the process.

Once a center asks to participate in the registry, the PI (principal investigator, the doctor that oversees the study) has to approve their participation because he is ultimately responsible for the conduct of the study no matter where it is being conducted. Once approved by PI, the IRB approval must be obtained for the investigators and the site. The IRB is the Institutional Review Board, a group of people (medical and non-medical) that reviews the study and consent form to make sure that the patient's rights are being protected. Most studies have to be IRB approved before you can enroll patients.

So, of course I wanted to know more about IRBs. Here's how the FDA government website defines them.

Under FDA regulations, an IRB is an appropriately constituted group that has been formally designated to review and monitor biomedical research involving human subjects. In accordance with FDA regulations, an IRB has the authority to approve, require modifications in (to secure approval), or disapprove research. This group review serves an important role in the protection of the rights and welfare of human research subjects.

The purpose of IRB review is to assure, both in advance and by periodic review, that appropriate steps are taken to protect the rights and welfare of humans participating as subjects in the research. To accomplish this purpose, IRBs use a group process to review research protocols and related materials (e.g., informed consent documents and investigator brochures) to ensure protection of the rights and welfare of human subjects of research.

Here we have another case of Medicare farming out the administrative tasks, in this case, reviewing the research studies. This new angle leads to the following exchange with Brittany Price about IRBs:

RF: Are IRBs registered with the FDA?
BP: IRBs are registered with the Office for Human Research Protections (OHRP), which is a government entity – not the FDA.

RF: Can anyone start one?
BP: If they meet the requirements.

RF: Does Provision have one, or plan to? If not, who do you use?
BP: No. We use multiple IRBs, including Copernicus Group Independent Review Board, Schulman Associates IRB, and CIRB.

RF: I presume you have a choice of IRBs?
BR: Yes, there are choices of IRBs.

RF: Can you shop around for the most favorable?
BP: Yes, to an extent. The study sponsor makes the decision of which IRB will oversee the study.

RF: Can you change IRBs?
BP: Yes, you can; however, that is not common during the study.

RF: Are they paid something for their work?
BP: Yes, they are paid for every submission, review and approval. They are paid by each site participating in the study.

RF: Can their decision be appealed?
BP: No. The IRB can make suggested changes or request further information, but their decision cannot be appealed.

After all of this information, we return to the subject of MACs, where the rubber meets the road. They must administer the payments. Again, Brittany Price explains.

MAC processes the claims for payment, not Medicare. It is their duty to review the claims for mistakes and determine if an office has done all it can to send a claim that is clean (free from charging mistakes or other errors in data) and payable (all codes meet criteria necessary to pass review and be paid). If there are any mistakes, they can send the claim back to the provider with a denial or can reject the claim from even processing if there are serious errors like code issues or Member ID number discrepancies. Although Medicare approves guidelines and LCD's, the MAC (Cahaba, for us) has the sole responsibility to review and process each claim looking both at Medicare's guidelines as well as the actual claim to be sure they are being good stewards of government money.

I never knew that Medicare involved itself in so many aspects of healthcare. Since the work of collecting the data gets handled by the party doing the research and MACs take care of the payments, Medicare can play a supervisory role.

I worry that its budget and resources may be endangered by current trends to downsize government expenditures from which we all benefit and would surely miss.

In the 2016 financial report for Provision, I noticed that 76% of the income for treatments came from Medicare. Perhaps this results from having a registry trial and drawing people whose insurance otherwise won't cover proton therapy, like me. I haven't seen the figures for other centers, so I can't compare.

The now defunct center in Indiana described problems collecting the proper amounts from Medicare and insurance companies as one cause of its downfall. Provision doesn't have that problem. Medicare and Provision came to my rescue when I was facing some drastic choices. I feel an obligation to present the availability of Medicare financing to as wide an audience as possible.

CHAPTER 15 Insurance

As a result of a study in 2009 by the American Society for Radiation Oncology (ASTRO) that suggested proton therapy isn't any better than less expensive alternatives, Aetna, United Healthcare, and Cigna stopped covering proton therapy for prostate cancer. Cigna announced proton therapy was not considered "medically necessary." That was quite a blow for both patients and the budding technology.

It comes as no surprise the report took that stand. The membership of ASTRO (more than 10,000) deals overwhelmingly with X-rays. It appears self-serving to find fault with a competing modality. To make things worse, the Journal of the National Cancer Institute then published a study saying proton therapy led to a modest reduction in side effects initially, but after one year was no different than IMRT. Since proton therapy usually costs significantly more than X-rays, insurance companies found a rationalization to deny coverage. However, Aetna did agree to cover those who were enrolled in clinical trials or registries!

In May, 2016, a whole edition of the Red Journal, a publication of ASTRO, was dedicated to proton therapy.

By clarifying the picture regarding the efficacy of proton therapy, these scholarly articles reversed the conclusion of the earlier article. Insurance companies, however, have not changed their stance despite the growing body of evidence.

With Medicare covering 80% of the cost of my proton therapy, United Healthcare agreed to pay the remaining twenty percent, subject to my annual out-of-pocket maximum of $4,900.

Then, Provision got United Healthcare to cover me in Knoxville as if I were in network, even though I was far from San Antonio. Thus, normal rates and co-pays pertained to a range of medical services.

Insurance companies require that a covered treatment be medically necessary, reasonable, appropriate, and evidence-based. How they interpret and apply these criteria vary considerably. A study conducted by M. D. Anderson published in March 2016 addressed this issue in Texas with the following conclusion:

Purpose: *The definition of medical necessity and indications for coverage of proton beam therapy (PBT) for the treatment of cancer can vary greatly among different professional societies (PSs) and payors. Variations in policies introduce substantial inefficiencies and limit access for patients who may clinically benefit from PBT. The purpose of this study was to analyze differences in medical necessity and coverage policies among payors and a PS.*
Results: *Proton beam therapy coverage in the state of Texas varied among payors and the PS for several disease sites, including the central nervous system, eyes, and prostate. The PS cited more references and higher levels of evidence than payor policies (P < .01). Levels of evidence were inconsistent between policies. Interestingly, only 18% to 29% of cited references overlapped between policies.*

A chart accompanying the study rated Aetna as the stingiest in providing coverage in Texas, followed closely by my insurance company, United Healthcare. When they deny coverage for proton therapy, hard decisions follow. Some men feel obliged to go ahead with surgery or other modalities that their insurance covers.

Others, however, pay for proton therapy out of their own pocket. Several years before Provision opened, one man in Knoxville mortgaged his home to go to Jacksonville, Florida, for proton therapy. Now, eight years later, he feels fine with no recurrence of the cancer. And, he still makes a monthly mortgage payment.

You can challenge the denial of coverage by your insurance company. I received much advice from Rhonda Turner at Provision about insurance. Below I excerpt some of her comments from the Provision blog.

"We believe it's important for patients to be empowered to fight for the coverage they deserve when facing a cancer diagnosis," says Rhonda Turner, manager of financial services at Provision Center for Proton Therapy. "We know that we won't always win every case, but together we can improve our chances for success."
Here's what financial services at Provision does to assist in the insurance process:

Letter of medical necessity and/or recommendation for treatment choice from other provider(s)
Peer-to-peer review calls
Individualized appeals
Multiple levels of appeals, including external reviews
Assist with patient appeal/grievance

Here's what patients can do to help:

File a patient grievance letter
Conference call with us and your insurer
Contact your employer—some employers can override insurance coverage decisions

Provision patients can also help in the fight for others, writing letters to insurance providers, sharing their stories on social media and contacting elected officials. "Public pressure is the best way to ensure coverage of proton therapy in the future," Turner says. "Nobody can communicate the need for proton

therapy better than those who are being denied access to it."
See more at: http://provisionproton.com/blog/page/2/#sthash.reFNLO3g.dpuf

What's the appropriate standard of evidence? Even the purveyors of proton therapy admit that it may take years to establish the kind of statistics being demanded.

I get pretty riled up about the rising costs of healthcare, driven by unconscionable prices and profits. Every other industrialized country in the world provides universal medical care for its citizens except for the United States. Their governments oversee the programs, including determining prices. Such a prospect meets stiff opposition here when people cry "socialism" and others insist on a free market approach. As a result, we pay twice the price and receive half the care.

Some writers get similarly worked up about the cost of proton therapy. On my blog website I have two long articles responding to what I feel are unjustified criticism of proton therapy. See: www.proton-beam-therapy.com/blog.html.

If insurance companies continue to resist, what can we do? A number of sources offer instruction, such as this Wall Street Journal article: http://www.proton-therapy.org/insurance_wsj_article.htm.

The National Association for Proton Therapy publishes a whole array of insurance strategies at http://www.proton-therapy.org/insurance_strategies.htm as well as a plethora of other information.

Another source is the Alliance for Proton Therapy Access, a nonprofit supported by the proton therapy industry. See: http://www.allianceforprotontherapy.org. I have an article about the Alliance, as well as another about criminal behavior on the part of insurance companies in denying coverage. See: http://www.proton-beam-therapy.com/blog.InsurersFightCancer.html and other articles.

The Alliance motto is: "Insurers: Fight Cancer, Not Me". A new national report found that more than 60 percent of adult cancer patients whose doctors prescribe proton therapy are initially denied by private insurers.

A new Alliance report – *Cancer Care Denied: The Broken State of Patient Access to Proton Therapy* – documents through patient stories and data the heavy emotional and financial burden cancer patients endure trying to get their insurer's approval for physician-recommended proton radiation therapy. Note, this isn't just a patient wanting it, but cases in which doctors recommend it.

The Alliance is calling on insurance commissioners in all 50 states to adopt and enforce the principles of a *Cancer Patients' Timely Treatment Bill of Rights* and hold insurers accountable for providing fair, timely, and transparent access to cancer treatment.

Adherents of proton therapy sometimes seek a political solution to insurance coverage. In Tennessee, after several years of effort on the part of the proton community, the legislature passed a bill specifying that state insurance companies had to cover proton therapy. However, the governor vetoed it. He was clearly in the pocket of the insurance lobby. Now they are trying to find the votes for an override.

In another instance, Oklahoma passed House Bill 1515 which prohibits health benefit plans from subjecting proton therapy to a higher standard of evidence than other types of radiation therapy when making coverage decisions. The House approved the legislation by a vote of 97-0. The bill's sponsor said:

Proton therapy went through several years of doing what they needed to and then the insurance companies took it and they were paying for it. For some reason now, they want them to go back and take several more years of testing. So they're trying to hold them to a higher standard than what they are with traditional radiation.

A proton therapy center in Hampton, Virginia, sued insurance companies for violating state laws in denying coverage. I guess the cost of the legal standoff is less than it would be to pay for the treatment, a cynical ploy.

After the insurance company denies coverage, a number of options exist to appeal and challenge that ruling. In the case of Medicare, it means dealing with yet another subcontractor. Google the phrase "medicare coverage appeal" and you will find four or five ads at the top of the page for companies that offer such services. The Medicare website describes the situation as follows.

First Level of Appeal: Redetermination by a Medicare Contractor

A redetermination is an examination of a claim by the Medicare Administrative Contractor (MAC) personnel who are different from the personnel who made the initial claim determination. The appellant (the individual filing the appeal) has 120 days from the date of receipt of the initial claim determination to file an appeal. The notice of initial determination is presumed to be received 5 days after the date of the notice unless there is evidence to the contrary. A redetermination must be requested in writing. A minimum monetary threshold is not required to request a redetermination.

Second Level of Appeal: Reconsideration by a Qualified Independent Contractor

A party to the redetermination may request a reconsideration if dissatisfied with the redetermination decision. A Qualified Independent Contractor (QIC) will conduct the reconsideration.

Filing a Request for Reconsideration

A written reconsideration request must be filed with a QIC within 180 days of receipt of the Medicare Redetermination Notice (MRN). The MRN is presumed to be received 5 days after the date of the notice unless there is evidence to the contrary. To request a reconsideration, follow the instructions on your MRN. A request for a reconsideration may be made on the standard form CMS-20033. To link to this form, scroll down to "Downloads". This form is mailed with the MRN. If the form is not used, the written request must contain all of the following information:

- Beneficiary's name
- Beneficiary's Medicare health insurance claim (HIC) number
- Specific service(s) and item(s) for which the reconsideration is requested, and the specific date(s) of service
- Name and signature of the party or representative of the party
- Name of the contractor that made the redetermination

The request should clearly explain why you disagree with the redetermination. A copy of the MRN and any other useful documentation should be sent with the reconsideration request to the appropriate QIC. Documentation that is submitted after the reconsideration request has been filed may result in an extension of the timeframe a QIC has to complete its decision. Further, the reconsideration request must contain any evidence noted in the redetermination as missing and any other evidence relevant to the appeal. However, it is not necessary to resubmit information that was already submitted to the contractor that made the redetermination. Evidence not submitted at the reconsideration level may be excluded from consideration at subsequent levels of appeal unless you show good cause for not submitting the evidence.

Besides the appeal process you can try to apply leverage in a different way. One man I met from Ohio fought Cigna tooth and nail for coverage to get proton therapy for his esophageal cancer, a condition for which the superiority of proton therapy is well established. It took five months and the intervention of his congressman before Cigna relented and he went to Provision for treatment. Unfortunately, by then, the cancer had metastasized to his bone. He passed away in January of 2017.

Cost is the leading issue for critics, not medical necessity or efficacy. What would be reasonable? How much should it cost? One source specifies Medicare coverage for proton therapy as being $1,200 per fraction. A different article says Medicare pays $841 for a session of proton therapy but only $411 for a session of X-rays. A third source claims IMRT costs about $16,000 whereas proton therapy rings in at $32,000. Yet another estimate marks fifty grand for proton therapy as being twice the cost of X-rays.

I know how much I personally paid, starting with my advantage HMO out-of-pocket copay of $4,819.72. The SpaceOAR added $3,015 more. Thus, I put $7,834.72 on my credit card.

Provision billed Medicare under code 77523 described as proton beam therapy delivery, intermediate level. Common practice seems to call for billing a higher amount than is likely to be paid. Provision then wrote off the portion of the billed amount not allowed by insurance. According to the forms I received in the mail from Medicare, Provision billed somewhat over $300,000 for my proton therapy and the various other fees and doctor visits. The best I can figure they ultimately received a little under $100,000.

My brother broke five ribs in a car accident. The total for his three-day hospital bill came to more than $60,000. Comparatively, my two months of treatment with protons were a bargain.

A number of proton therapy centers, including the University of Pennsylvania, the University of Maryland, and the two Mayo Clinics, charge the same for proton therapy as for X-rays. You would think in response to such pricing insurance companies would be more willing to pay for proton therapy, but the Maryland center tells me they still get hassled about medical necessity.

Thomas R. Bortfeld and Jay S. Loeffler have written:

And in the United States, major insurance companies are denying proton therapy . . . on the basis that there are too few rigorously designed and completed clinical trials providing evidence of better outcomes. In our experience, however, this is a vicious cycle: such trials are difficult to conduct when patients are denied private health coverage[5].
(See: https://www.nature.com/news/three-ways-to-make-proton-therapy-affordable-1.22660)

In some cases, the cost for the initial treatment is equal to or less than that of X-rays. M. D. Anderson Cancer Center reports this to be true for accelerated partial breast treatment, as follows:

A new study by MD Anderson Cancer Center reveals that proton therapy is a cost-effective treatment for early-stage breast cancer, compared to other therapies.The study found that the cost of proton therapy when used for accelerated partial breast irradiation (to decrease overall treatment time and toxicity) was estimated at $13,833. By comparison, intensity-modulated radiation therapy (X-rays) for whole breast irradiation was $19,599.
(For more information, see https://www.mdanderson.org/patients-family/diagnosis-treatment/care-centers-clinics/proton-therapy-center.html.)

Perhaps these figures would convince an insurance company, which is concerned more with the bottom line than with healing cancer. Even when the cost is lower, insurance companies have balked at payment, perhaps feeling their cost avoidance would be exposed.

I frequently receive emails from people asking how they can get proton therapy when their insurance company is resistant. Here's what I tell them.

1. Fight back. You will need the assistance of your doctor and perhaps other professionals. At Provision they have seven people working full-time in the insurance department. On the other hand, I was not very pleased with M. D. Anderson. They are so huge and so famous that they are swamped with

business. They don't really need your business and may not be aggressive in helping you. When I told them United Healthcare wouldn't cover proton therapy for prostate cancer, the person on the phone said "I'm sorry." Provision, on the other hand, led me to a registry.

2. Are you old enough to be on Medicare? If so, you can be in a registry, as I was, which will result in Medicare paying 80% of the cost, whether or not your insurance company covers it. For me, once Medicare paid 80%, United Healthcare agreed to pay the other 20%.

3. Shop around for cost. I asked the proton center at the University of Florida in Jacksonville the cost for my proton therapy for prostate cancer. They said $134,000. When I asked the same question of Provision, they said $93,000, for the very same treatment. Actually, better, as their equipment is more advanced.

4. A few proton centers charge the same for proton therapy as for X-rays. This is true, I believe, for the two Mayo Clinic centers (Phoenix AZ and Rochester MN), the University of Pennsylvania, and the University of Maryland centers. Perhaps if proton therapy didn't cost so much more than X-rays, more insurance companies would approve treatment.

5. Go abroad. If you are paying for treatment yourself, it is cheaper to go abroad. Another insurance strategy might be to help the insurance company by finding the least expensive proton treatment. In that way, you could be allies rather than adversaries.

Authors Thomas R. Bortfeld and JayS. Loeffler suggest the following:

> *Insurance companies should move to the 'reference pricing' model, which establishes a common level of payment for different therapies that have similar anticipated outcomes[10]. This will help to build the evidence for the benefit of proton therapy (or lack of it) in new clinical applications. The Mayo Clinic in Rochester, Minnesota, has already entered into such arrangements with insurers.*
> *(See: https://www.nature.com/news/three-ways-to-make-proton-therapy-affordable-1.22660)*

We're not alone in facing issues with insurance coverage for proton therapy. In England, where they have universal healthcare, the National Health Service (NHS) determines treatments and pays for them. Or not. Their reluctance to approve proton therapy has led to several celebrated cases. One was Alex Vincent, who as a young child was diagnosed with a brain tumor. Doctors at the NHS gave him an 80% likelihood of dying, and even if he survived, conventional treatment may have left him blind, deaf, and in a wheelchair. As Alex was only four years old, X-rays would have caused serious damage to his still developing body.

Even before the diagnosis, Alex's father went to the internet for independent advice. He found his son's symptoms were consistent with brain tumor. Only when he took his son to a different hospital did a scan confirm a tumor. Then, he went back to the internet. He tells his story:

"I remember in 2008, googling 'anaplastic ependymoma' and I found this link to a hospital in Massachusetts, offering proton beam therapy. It said on the link it was the way forward for babies, toddlers and small children. So I told the specialist in Britain I wanted to take Alex to America for proton therapy treatment rather than having radiotherapy here. He just said: 'It isn't tried and tested.' He warned us that if we took Alex to the States, we were putting his life in danger. Then he added: 'And anyway, they are probably only after your money.' But I just stuck to my guns."

After the family scrambled to raise the money, Alex was treated in the United States, first surgery, then proton therapy (received in Jacksonville, Florida). His father reports:

"While we were in Florida, all the things the British doctors had told me proton therapy wasn't good for – all these different tumours – actually, it turned out, could be treated with it. The doctors here in the UK had said it was only good for tumours at the base of the back of the neck. That wasn't the case. The proton treatment is good for lots of different tumours."

Today Alex is a rambunctious young man in excellent health, no thanks to the NHS. The family founded an inspiring website called Alex's Lemonade Stand Foundation, named after one of the activities for raising money. See: https://www.alexslemonade.org/childhood-cancer/type/brain-tumor.

A more recent case involves Ashya King, also with a brain tumor, also given poor advice by the NHS. I tell the story at the end of this book in my book review.

The NHS has now paid for some one hundred cases of pediatric cancers to be treated by proton therapy (at an average cost of more than $100,000 each), but it remains an on-going battle. What stands out in my mind is the terrible advice that the doctors gave in their evaluation of proton therapy, and how wrong they were. Only by bucking the system, at great personal and financial expense, were these parents able to save their children's lives. How many parents are capable of doing the same?

I have stressed that I am not giving medical advice in this book. That should be left to the medical establishment. Unfortunately, many times they give poor advice, as we have seen. By knowing more ourselves, we are better qualified to determine whether the doctor's advice fits our needs.

CHAPTER 16 FUTURE CONSIDERATIONS

After starting slowly, the building of proton therapy centers has reached a high pitch of activity, both in the United States and around the world.

While I present proton therapy as fighting resistance from the medical community, don't think for a moment that it's in any way "alternative." This new competition with X-rays is coming firmly from within the establishment. At Provision CARES Proton Therapy Center in Knoxville, Tennessee, where I was treated, the proton center is part of a much larger practice that includes chemotherapy, X-rays, and other mainstream modalities. They do trials for Big Pharma. The doctors do not hesitate to prescribe drugs. I don't get along well with medicine for profit, but I sure do like protons.

Provision is unique in that they formed a sister company, ProNova, to manufacture proton therapy equipment. They are on the leading edge of improving pencil beam scanning and superconducting technology. My wife Linda and I toured their very impressive facility.

Superconducting magnets must be powerful to bend the proton beam and control its direction. At ProNova workers wind the magnets onsite and then encase them in highly insulated containers in which they lower the temperature to three degrees Kelvin (about 450 degrees below zero Fahrenheit). The outer shell remains at room temperature. The low temperature effectively reduces electrical resistance to almost nil. Otherwise the massive current would cause high heat and require enormous amounts of electricity.

ProNova's superconducting magnets draw four watts! Four! (Compare to a 60-watt light bulb.) Cyclotrons typically require outrageous amounts of electricity, with electrical bills approaching a million dollars a year. Now, superconducting cyclotrons are under development. They will be smaller, easier to transport, and far more efficient.

Established suppliers of proton equipment include IBA, Varian and Mevion. If you are interested in this technology, you may want to look at their websites. ProNova and a company called ProTom International join this elite group.

Imaging is an important part of proton therapy. You must be able to accurately identify and locate the tumor. Hence, MRI, CT scans, and X-rays are essential to the treatment. New equipment often includes cone beam imaging built right into the proton equipment.

ProTom International is developing proton tomography, a far more accurate type of imaging that uses protons rather than X-rays. For this purpose, they use 350 Mev, which requires a synchrotron. Other companies, including Mevion, are also looking into proton imaging.

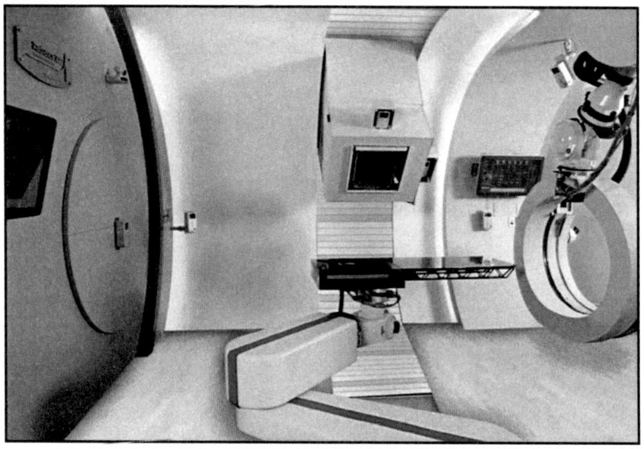

The Radiance 330 system by ProTom.

The first ProTom installation is being completed at Massachusets General Hospital in Boston even as I write this. It has no huge gantry and requires a much smaller area and less shielding. As a result, it's being built into an existing space formerly occupied by two LINAC machines (X-rays). This reduces the cost to a very manageable level. In my communications with ProTom, I have been impressed by the potential of their technology.

Other companies are constantly upgrading their technology, as well. For example, the following press release from IBA summarizes the current state of their equipment:

> *The Proteus®PLUS . . . is configured with two gantry treatment rooms equipped with IBA's pencil beam scanning (PBS) and Cone Beam Computed Tomography (CBCT) large field of view image guidance. These technologies improve the precision of treatment and enable adaptive treatment. The center also benefits from the most advanced room matching available, enabling maximum flexibility of room scheduling and allowing for a minimum 30% reduction in commissioning time therefore giving maximum flexibility for patient treatment. Rooms are also supplied with IBA's wireless hand pendant, the only wireless patient remote control in the radiation therapy industry as well as a new generation, high accuracy and precision Patient Positioning System.*
> *(IBA has an interesting website at https://iba-worldwide.com/proton-therapy.)*

Disclosure: I own some IBA stock. To be honest, it hasn't done that well.

Mevion has developed a single room configuration which it believes will meet the current market. In their description, they make a little dig, saying none of the centers with their equipment have gone bankrupt. The financial failures all came from the large multi-room centers which may have bitten off more than they could chew.

Several centers that have the earlier S250 model from Mevion are expanding to get the newer version with Hyperscan pencil beam scanning capability. In their promotional videos they make two claims to being unique. First, they have the fastest switching between layers. Secondly, they have introduced a multi-leaf collimator (MLC) to shape the proton beams laterally. The MLC technology has long been used with X-rays. Adding it to the proton arsenal can help to improve its accuracy.

According to Wikipedia an MLC is a device made up of individual "leaves" of a high atomic numbered material, usually tungsten, that can move independently in and out of the path of a particle beam in order to block it. Shaping the beam has been done with apertures in proton therapy, but they must be custom made for each individual client.

I requested permission to use a graph on Mevion's website that showed the increase in demand for single-room systems, but they denied my request. So I sent the following email:

> *Thanks for responding. I'm a little confused, especially since you are involved in marketing, that you don't want me to include this information about Mevion in my book. I mention IBA, ProNova, Varian and ProTom as well. If you would rather have me not include Mevion, I will honor your request, but I just want to clarify that is your intention.*

To which I received the following reply:

> *There are considerable regulations about how we directly promote or endorse the clinical efficacy of proton therapy. We don't feel comfortable with the tacit endorsement to this use without much closer regulatory review. Thank you for considering us for your book.*

I appreciate their principled stand. They probably would think that I have far over-sold proton therapy in this book and made unproven claims as to its efficacy. That's why I like the proton center in Prague. They don't qualify their claims with "may" or "sometimes." They just tell it as they see it. I am doing the same thing. I am writing from a patient's point of view, not a scientific paper.

Varian also made a very principled statement in a press release which I quote here at length:

> *Statements in this press release regarding future business, plans, objectives, expectations and other similar matters; market acceptance of products or technology for proton therapy; timing and ability to achieve certain results; and any statements using the terms "enables," "offers," "can," "feasible," and "will," are forward-looking statements that involve risks and uncertainties*

that could cause actual results to differ materially from those anticipated.

These risks and uncertainties include demand for the company's proton therapy products; the company's ability to develop and commercialize new proton therapy products; the company's ability to meet regulatory regulations or procedures; the company's ability to protect the company's intellectual property; and the other risks listed from time to time in the company's filings with the Securities and Exchange Commission, which by this reference are incorporated herein.

These forward-looking statements represent the Company's judgment as of the date of this press release. The Company assumes no obligation to update or revise these forward-looking statements because of new information, future events, or otherwise.

This kind of caution is called due diligence and it is essential in financial dealings. I laud them for the stance they are taking. Perhaps some of the centers that have been having financial difficulties could have benefitted from such an approach.

Considering Mevion's statement about the high demand of single-room proton centers, and considering that all of the other manufacturers produce a similar product, I looked at the list of proton centers currently in the planning or building stage. There are sixteen centers on the list, and five of them are getting single-room centers, of which none happen to be Mevion. Three are Varian, one IBA, and one yet to be determined.

A number of companies have announced plans to build more proton centers. Provision is building centers in western Tennessee and in Orlando, Florida. Their long-term goal is to open fifteen centers. Meanwhile, I found the following in a news release from Providence, a company developing a proton center in Birmingham, Alabama:

Providence Proton Therapy was formed to develop proton therapy cancer treatment centers where they are currently not available, thereby helping cancer patients and local communities. Our goal is to create ten proton therapy centers throughout the United States. Our initial concentration is within the Southeast. Our purpose and desired outcome is unique in terms of developing proton therapy centers in that we are attempting to custom design the structure of each center and the relationship with a local strategic partner to uniquely fit the needs of the strategic partner and community. In other words, we do not take a "cookie-cutter" or "one size fits all" approach.

(See http://providenceprotontherapy.com/.)

Pardon me for being a bit amused by their assumptions. They want to put proton centers where there aren't any, yet another one is being planned for Birmingham by a different company. And "cookie cutter"? Really? Is there a company just stamping out proton therapy centers? Who?

Another similarly named company, Provident, which took over the difficult situation at Emory

University in Atlanta, plans another three centers, one of which will be in Baton Rouge.

In an article called "Three Ways to Make Proton Therapy Affordable," authors Thomas R. Bortfeld and Jay S. Loeffler from Massachusetts General Hospitals's proton therapy center suggest these areas for improvement:

1. Shrink accelerators. They are doing this at Mass General with their new ProTom International installation.

2. Sharpen beams. This refers to PBS as preferred over double-scattering. They make this point: "(proton) therapy is not like a pill: its success depends on how it is delivered. It has more room for improvement than other, more established radiation treatments, such as X-rays."

3. Broaden healthcare coverage. This is indeed essential. In their article they make a very concise case for protons, which I quote below.

If cost was not an issue, proton therapy would be the treatment of choice for most patients with localized tumours. Protons can be targeted more precisely than X-rays, so the tissues around the tumour receive two to three times less radiation. This lowers the chance of causing secondary tumours or impairing white blood cells and the immune system. High doses of protons can be delivered safely to hard-to-treat tumours: for instance, those at the base of the skull or in the liver. Such accuracy is crucial when treating cancers in children.

From the same article:

Three developments that have emerged in the past three years hold promise. Narrow 'pencil' beams that paint the radiation dose precisely onto a tumour reduce the need to treat patients from many angles. Rapid imaging methods can detect tiny changes in the patient's position, so that the beam can be shifted. And advanced 'soft robotics' built using malleable outer materials will soon allow patients to be positioned quickly and comfortably using robotic hands.
(See: https://www.nature.com/news/three-ways-to-make-proton-therapy-affordable-1.22660)

Not surprisingly, many proton therapy companies are turning toward the burgeoning market in China. They aren't alone according to this description from *China Particle Therapy News*.

Backed by rich private investors, proton therapy, a highly precise but expensive form of radiation used to treat cancer, is booming in China. The country has gone from having no operating proton therapy centers two and a half years ago to having two in operation today plus at least 43 more proton projects in various stages of development.

Rather than stemming from demand from the medical community, this building spree in China originates from the country's shifting economic winds. Chinese investors have seen returns from traditionally lucrative stakes in manufacturing and real estate decline in recent years, and that has made *investment in medical centers, particularly ones focused on a cutting-edge technology, an area of increasing popularity, says Yu Hongxia, general manager of APH Medical, a subsidiary of a medical supplies company that is investing 1.6 billion yuan ($240 million) in a proton center in southeastern China.*

Further encouraging this interest is a 2015 decision by the government to relax restrictions on the importing of medical equipment. That made it easy to purchase proton-beam systems from foreign manufacturers.

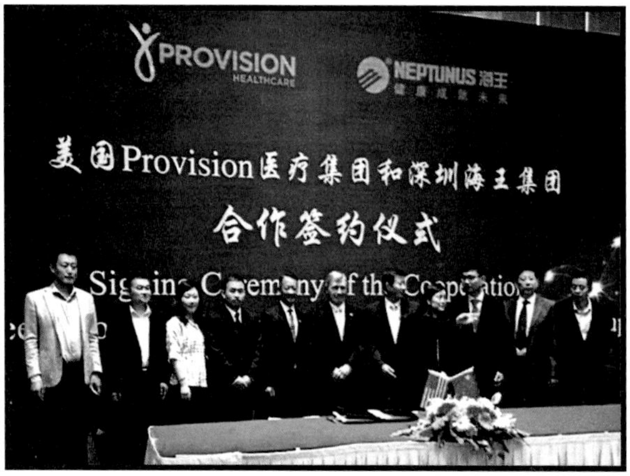

One center in Shanghai promotes medical tourism for proton therapy to prospective patients from the United States. I question the accuracy of their assessment.

In the US, patients need to wait for 4 months in making appointment for Proton Beam Therapy, and cost them $150,000. In Shanghai, patients may have the same quality of treatment without waiting period, and cost only for $50,000. Contact the China Medical Tourism Inc. at SHANGHAI's Center of Proton Therapy: info@shmtppp.com.

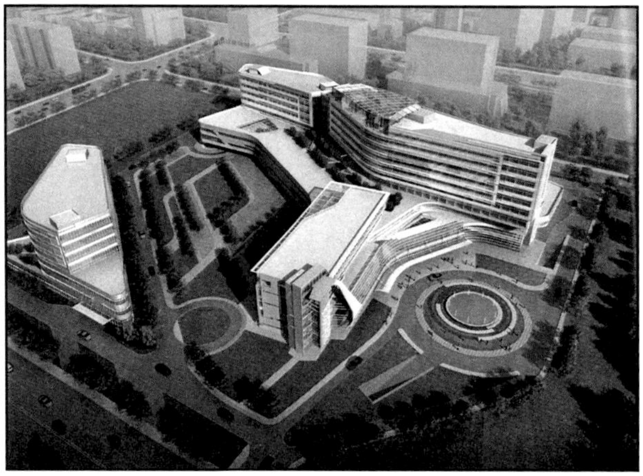

Beside this proposed one-thousand bed hospital in China, the empty field in the upper left is reserved for the Provision CARES Proton Therapy Center.

I have been told that China is three times our size with twice the rate of cancer, which means a market six times that in the United States. Here, our five-year survival rate for all cancers is 70% but in China it's only 30%. No wonder they want forty proton therapy centers. Provision has already arranged for some partnerships there.

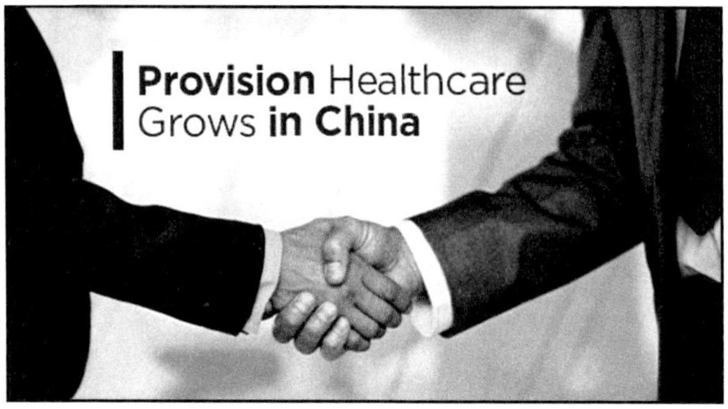

Such rapid expansion of proton therapy centers elicits another concern, namely, the availability of qualified and experienced workers. Many of the people I met at Provision have worked at other proton therapy centers, in Florida or Oklahoma or elsewhere.

Where will all of these centers find staff? Greg Sonnenfeld, director of Shreveport's Willis-Knighton Cancer Center, has said recruiting and retaining specialists well versed in the technology has been a struggle. There has been a lot of moving from one center to another. For example, my doctor at Provision, Mario Fagundes, a leader in the field, left to go to the new center in Miami (closer to family and his native Brazil). The proton center in Dallas enticed Dr. Andrew K. Lee, a leading proton therapy expert and one of the founders of proton therapy at M. D. Anderson, to become their Medical Director. He was the first physician to treat patients with pencil beam scanning and pioneered the use of fiducial markers. I can see how he might be attracted to a new center with the latest technology.

Former executives from ProCure, which founded several proton therapy centers, left to form Proton International, a full-service design and management company for proton therapy centers, specializing in one- and two-room treatment facilities.

As more and more centers open, it won't work to simply try to attract experts from other centers. For that reason, Provision has an extensive training program. Then, much like a sous chef at a fine restaurant moving on to open his or her own restaurant, after they get some experience, proton workers go into the market place to find more lucrative opportunities.

The University of Florida addresses this need. All of the staff at the Proton Therapy Institute are faculty members at the university, where they train the next generation of proton therapy workers. If I were a young doctor or radiology technician, I would definitely become involved with proton therapy, an exciting field with great job security.

The equipment manufacturer Varian and the University of Pennsylvania Proton Therapy Center have joined together to provide a 40-week training program in all aspects of proton therapy, combined with onsite internships. They offer to give their training at other proton centers, as well. So, some steps are being taken to meet the need.

Another possibility is for personnel experienced with X-rays to switch to protons. Since both involve radiation, many of the procedures are the same. If X-ray practitioners are feeling threatened by proton therapy, why not jump ship. As you can gather from this chapter, proton therapy is where the action is right now. Why not join the crowd?

Appendix

Final words

I have a little more to include here, in the spirit of a memoir, for which I could find no place within the text.

In 2001 my then-wife, Ruth, was diagnosed with breast cancer. For five years we chose alternative therapies (including going to a clinic in Germany) at a personal cost of almost $40,000 a year (insurance didn't cover them), adding up to $200,000, which was half of my income at the time. In the end, after we decided to go conventional with chemo and radiation, Ruth was dead within a year. The treatment itself was her demise, not the cancer. At Provision, they treat breast cancer. How I wish it had been possible for my Ruthie to get proton therapy. She died in January of 2007.

At the time, I discounted any possibility of another relationship. Six months later, however, I met Linda. We stayed in touch until I was ready and got married (on a labyrinth) in June of 2010. Our courtship and love affair has been closely tied to cruise ships and transatlantic voyages. I wrote a memoir about our love story, called *Cruise of the Heart: Memoir of a Transatlantic Voyage*. It is for the cruise industry much like what this book is for proton beam therapy.

I did the final editing and proofing of the first edition of this book while on a three-week cruise from Tampa, Florida, to Vancouver, British Columbia, in April of 2017. The full-service environment (room cleaned, meals provided) gave me plenty of time to write. Of course Linda remained here by my side, working on a photography and poetry book of her own.

During my twenty plus years as a professional labyrinth maker, I have written a number of instructional and informational books available on Amazon.com, including the following:

The Labyrinth Revival: A Personal Account
Constructing the Chartres Labyrinth
Constructing Classical Labyrinths
Canvas Labyrinths Construction Manual
Church Labyrinths
Origin, Symbolism and Design of the Chartres Labyrinth

I have a number of websites, where you can find out information on proton therapy and more about me:

www.labyrinth-enterprises.com
www.robertferre.com
www.cruiseoftheheart.com
www.retiredgonecruising.com
www.protontherapybook.com
www.proton-beam-therapy.com
www.proton-therapy-centers.com

Websites of interest

ackermancancer.com
A private clinic in Jacksonville, FL, with proton therapy, on the registry with Provision.

biomed-research.com
The research division of Provision Healthcare.

bryant-research.com/html/about.html
Bryant Research, a report on Proton Therapy.

clinicaltrials.gov
List of clinical trials.

emma.msrb.org/IssueView/IssueDetails.aspx?id=EA352368
EMMA Electronic Municipal Market Access website to check the status of any proton therapy center financed with public bonds.

livestrong.com
Cancer information.

prayasyougo.com
A daily devotion by a Jesuit group in London.

proton-beam-therapy.com
My proton blog.

proton-cancer-treatment.com
English-language website for the proton therapy center in Prague. They are quite convinced they are the leading proton therapy center in the world.

proton-therapy.org
The National Association for Proton Therapy. Includes a ton of information.

proton-therapy-today.com
An online magazine about proton therapy.

protonbob.com/about-proton-therapy/proton-therapy-myths
Debunks myths about proton therapy.

protontherapybook.com
The website associated with this and my other proton therapy book(s). It contains full-color photos and illustrations, including some that are not in the books.

allianceforprotontherapy.org
A nonprofit organization supported by the proton therapy industry to encourage insurance coverage and report cases, both positive and negative.

ptcog.ch
The Particle Therapy Co-Operative Group.

texascenterforprotontherapy.com
Proton therapy center on the same Medicare registry with Provision.

Use of material from the internet

Section 107 of the Copyright Act states: "The fair use of a copyrighted work, including such use by reproduction in copies or phonograph records or by any other means specified by that section, for purposes such as criticism, comment, news reporting, teaching (including multiple copies for classroom use), scholarship, or research, is not an infringement of copyright." I consider this book to be research. I have done my best to attribute photos and illustrations. If I have used anything that the owner would like me to remove, please let me know.

Contact information

As a proton therapy ambassador, I'm ready and willing to give presentations, answer questions, or otherwise spread the word.

Robert Ferré
Email: robert@protontherapybook.com

Many people made this book better by contributing content, teaching me, directing me to relevant sources, making suggestions, proofreading, providing illustrations, and many other ways. My heartfelt thanks to all of you.

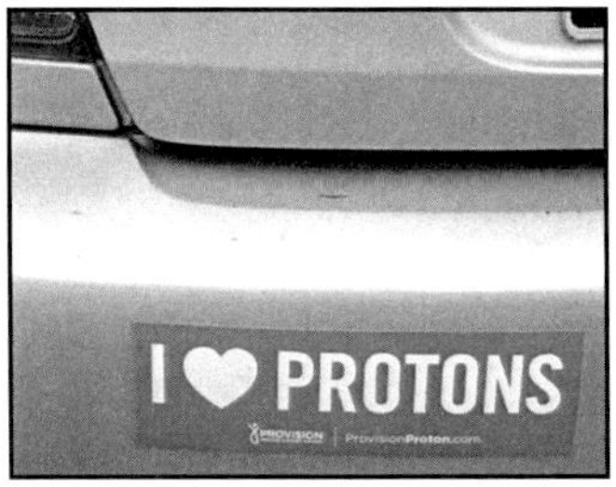

My bumper sticker. People unfamiliar with proton therapy may be a bit puzzled. Now, you know.

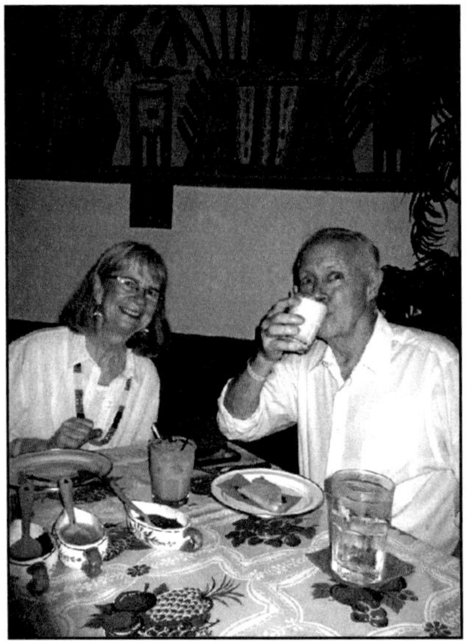

Linda and me in Mexico in January, 2017. I was fully recovered. In April we took a celebratory cruise through the Panama Canal.

Proton Therapy Centers in the United States

This list does not include low-energy centers that treat only ocular cancer. The abbreviations are as follows: G = Gantry, F = Fixed beam (including those that can move up to 60%), PBS = pencil beam scanning.

Name/Contact/Affiliation	Open	#Room	Contact Information	#PBS	Comments
CENTERS IN OPERATION					
ARIZONA					
Mayo Clinic Proton Beam Therapy Center 5881 E, Mayo Boulevard Phoenix, AZ 85054	2016	4G	480.369-5200 www.mayoclinic.org/departments-centers/proton-beam-therapy-program/sections/proton-therapy-facilities/gnc-20187682	4	Doing a trial comparing IMRT and proton therapy.
CALIFORNIA					
James M. Slater, M.D. Proton Treatment and Research Center 11234 Anderson Street Loma Linda, CA 92354	1990	3G 1F	800.PROTONS (800.776.8667) www.protons.com	?	Treated more than 20,000 patients. Has published the longest-term clinical outcomes. Got best website address and 800 number.
California Protons Cancer Therapy Center 9730 Summers Ridge Rd. San Diego, CA 92121	2014	3G 2F	858.549.7400 www.californiaprotons.com	5	All five treatment rooms have pencil beam scanning. New ownership and management, December, 2017.
FLORIDA					
Ackerman Cancer Center 10881 San Jose Boulevard Jacksonville, FL 32223	2015	1G	904.880.5522 ackermancancercenter.com/proton-therapy/what-is-proton-therapy/	1	First private physician-funded proton center in the United States. Mevion S250 equipment.

Name/Contact/Affiliation	Open	#Room	Contact Information	#PBS	Comments
The Marjorie and Leonard Williams Center for Proton Therapy, U of Florida Health Center at Orlando Health 1400 S. Orange Avenue Orlando, FL 32806	2016	1G	321.841.8650 www.ufhealthcancer orlando.com/centers/ proton-therapy-center	1	Soon Provision will be opening a second proton therapy center in Orlando. Within a few years Florida will have six centers.
U of Florida Proton Therapy Institute 2015 N. Jefferson Street Jacksonville, FL 32206	2006	3G 1F	904.588.1800 www.floridaproton.org	0	2018 expansion planned to get pencil beam scanning
Miami Cancer Institute at Baptist Health South 8900 N. Kendall Drive Miami, FL 33176	2018	3 G	786.527.8010, 786.596.2000 www.baptisthealth.net/en/ lp/pages/miami-cancer-institute.aspx	3	Part of a large cancer institute.
ILLINOIS					
Northwestern Medicine Chicago Proton Center 4455 Weaver Parkway Warrenville, IL 60555 (Chicago)	2010	1G 3F	877.887.5807 www.cdhprotoncenter.com www.chicagoprotoncenter .com	?	Chicago area.
LOUISIANA					
Willis-Knighton Proton Therapy Center 2600 Kings Highway Shreveport, LA 71103	2014	1G	318.212.8300 www.wkhs.co/Cancer/ Cancer-Treatment-Services/Proton-Therapy	1	First to use the IBA ProteousOne single treatment room equipment.
MARYLAND					
Maryland Proton Treatment Center University of Maryland 850 West Baltimore Street, Baltimore, MD 21201	2016	4G 1F	410.369.5200 www.mdproton.com	5	Charges the same for proton therapy as for regular X-rays. That should make it more available for insurance coverage. Equipment by Varian.
MASSACHUSETTS					
Francis H. Burr Proton Therapy Center Massachusetts General Hospital, 30 Fruit Street Boston, MA 02114	2003	2G 1F	617.726.0923 Inquiries: 617.724.1680 www.massgeneral.org/ radiationoncology/ BurrProtonCenter.aspx		2018 expansion with ProTom International treatment room in two former LINAC rooms.

Name/Contact/Affiliation	Open	#Room	Contact Information	#PBS	Comments
MICHIGAN					
Proton Therapy Center at Beaumont Hospital Cancer Ctr. 3601 W. Thirteen Mile Road Royal Oak, MI 48073	2017	1G	248.551.8402 www.beaumont.org/treatments/proton-therapy	1	IBA ProteusOne
MINNESOTA					
Mayo Clinic Proton Beam Therapy Center 190 Second Street NW Rochester, MN 55901	2015	4G	507.284.2511 www.mayoclinic.org/departments-centers/proton-beam-therapy-program/sections/proton-therapy-facilities/gnc-20187682	4	Conducting clinical trials on proton therapy.
MISSOURI					
S. Lee Kling Proton Therapy Center Barnes-Jewish Hospital, St. Louis, MO	2013	1G	314.286.1222 www.siteman.wustl.edu/treatment/siteman-approach/radiation/proton-beam-therapy/	0	The center houses the compact Mevion S250™ Proton Beam Therapy System. Part of the Siteman Cancer Center.
NEW JERSEY					
The Laurie Proton Therapy Center at Robert Wood Johnson University Hospital, One Robert Wood Johnson Place New Brunswick, NJ 08901	2015	1G	888.MD.RWJUH (888.637.9584) www.rwjuh.edu/proton-therapy/proton-therapy.aspx	1	Midway between New York and Philadelphia. Mevion S250.
ProCure Proton Therapy Center 103 Cedar Grove Lane Somerset, NJ 08873	2012	4G	877.967.7628 www.procure.com/New-Jersey-Explore	0	One of several ProCure facilities.
OHIO					
Cincinnati Children's Proton Therapy Center 7777 Yankee Road Liberty Township, OH 45044	2016	3G	877.881.8479 www.cincinnatichildrens.org	3	One gantry dedicated to research only. Room for a fourth gantry.

Name/Contact/Affiliation	Open	#Room	Contact Information	#PBS	Comments
University Hospitals Seidman Cancer Center 11100 Euclid Avenue Cleveland, OH 44106	2016	1G	866.UH4.CARE (844.2273) www.uhhospitals.org/seidman/services/radiation-oncology/our-technology/proton-therapy	1	Mevion S250.
OKLAHOMA					
ProCure Proton Therapy Center 5901 W. Memorial Road Oklahoma City, OK 73142	2009	1G 3F	888.847.2640 www.procure.com/Oklahoma-Explore	0	Largest of the two proton centers in Oklahoma City.
Stephenson Cancer Center Proton Center at the U of Oklahoma, 800 NE 10th Street Oklahoma City, OK 73104	2015	1G	855.750.2273 www.oumedicine.com/cancer	0	Very dense website with little information about proton therapy. Mevion S250.
PENNSYLVANIA					
Roberts Proton Therapy Center University of Pennsylvania Penn Medicine 3400 Civic Center Boulevard Philadelphia, PA 19104	2010	4G 1F	800.789.7366 www.pennprotontherapy.org	0	Very busy. Offer training to the proton therapy industry. Building a new proton therapy center in New Jersey. Calls itself the largest proton therapy center in the world.
TENNESSEE					
Provision CARES Proton Therapy Center Knoxville 6450 Provision Cares Way Knoxville, TN 37909	2014	2G 1F + 1G 1F	865.862.1600 www.provisionproton.com	5	Three treatment rooms with IBA equipment, two with new ProNova equipment (2018)
St. Jude Red Frog Events Proton Therapy Center 262 Danny Thomas Place Memphis, TN 38105	2015	2G 1F	866.278.5833 www.stjude.org/treatment/services/radiation-oncology/proton-therapy.html	3	Children only. Named after an events promotion company that raised millions for the center.
TEXAS					
M. D. Anderson Proton Therapy Center 1840 Old Spanish Trail Houston, TX 77054	2006	3G 1F	866.632.4782 www.mdanderson.org/patients-family/diagnosis-treatment/care-centers-clinics/proton-therapy-center.html	?	Why such an unwieldy website? Pioneered pencil beam scanning.

Name/Contact/Affiliation	Open	#Room	Contact Information	#PBS	Comments
Texas Center for Proton Therapy 1501 West Royal Lane Irving, TX 75063	2015	2G 1F	469.513.5500 www.texascenterforproton therapy.com	3	Joining Medicare registry for proton therapy with Provision and Ackerman
VIRGINIA					
Hampton University Proton Therapy Institute 40 Enterprise Parkway Hampton, VA 23666	2010	4G 1F	757.251.6800 www.hamptonproton.org	0	Claims to be the largest free-standing proton therapy center (until New York City's center is completed).
WASHINGTON					
ProCure SCCA Proton Therapy Center 1570 North 115th Street Seattle WA 98133	2013	4G 1F or 1G 2F	877.897.7628 www.sccaprotontherapy .com	?	SCCA = Seattle Cancer Care Alliance .
WASHINGTON D.C.					
Georgetown Lombardi Comprehensive Cancer Center at Medstar Georgetown University Hospital 3800 Reservoir Road N.W. Washington D.C. 20057	2018	1G	855.546.2805 www.medstargeorgetown. org/our-services/cancer-care/treatments/proton-beam-therapy/	1	Second center soon to open in Washington D.C.
CENTERS UNDER CONSTRUCTION OR PLANNED					
ALABAMA					
Providence Proton Center St. Vincent's Birmingham 1200 Corporate Drive, Suite 470 Birmigham, AL 35242	2019	1G	Jame Curtis: 205.451.7839 www.providenceprotonther apy.com	1	IBA single gantry
ALABAMA					
University of Alabama at Birmingham		1G	PR dept: 205-934-3884	1	Developed by Proton International.

Name/Contact/Affiliation	Open	#Room	Contact Information	#PBS	Comments
FLORIDA					
Delray Radiation Therapy Center 5352 Linton Avenue Delray Beach, FL 33484	2018	1G		1G	Developed by Proton International Opening scheduled for 2018.
The Sylvester Comprehensive Cancer Care at the University of Miami Miller School of Medicine 1475 NW 12th Avenue Miami, FL 33136	2020	1G	305.699.6417 www.umiamihealth.org/Sylvester	1	Will be the second center in Miami.
Provision CARES Proton Therapy Center Orlando, Florida	2020	2G 1F		3	Has been delayed.
GEORGIA					
Georgia Proton Therapy Center 615 Peachtree Street NE Atlanta, GA 30308	2019	4G 1F	707.217.7565 www.georgiaproton.com	5	Project taken over by new owners with massive debt.
LOUISIANA					
Louisiana Proton Care Center Baton Rouge					Developed by Provident Proton Care, a division of Provident Resource Group, Baton Rouge, LA
MICHIGAN					
The McLaren Proton Therapy Center G-4100 Beecher Road Flint, MI 48532	M	3G	855.697.7686	3	Original vendor went bankrupt. New developer installing Russian-made equipment. Not certain this is a viable project.
NEW JERSEY					
Virtua Voorhees Hospital 100 Bowman Drive Voorhees Township, NJ 08043	2020	1	856.247.3000 www.virtua.org/news/proton-therapy-to-south-jersey	1	Being developed by the University of Pennsylvania Penn Medicine. Varian equipment.
NEW YORK					
New York Proton Regional Center		4 + 1	212-268-3165 or maybe 212.751.8337		250,000 sq. ft. facility. Varian equipment. Four treatment rooms, plus one for research.

Name/Contact/Affiliation	Open	#Room	Contact Information	#PBS	Comments
755 2nd Avenue New York, NY 10017			www.nyprc.com www.newyorkprotoncenter .com		
NORTH CAROLINA					
Duke University Health System Durham, NC	2020	2G		2	Developed by Provision Cares Proton Therapy ProNova equipment.
TENNESSEE					
Provision CARES Proton Therapy Nashville 4588 Carothers Pkwy. Franklin, TN 37067	2018	2G 1F	844.742.2737 www.nashvilleproton.com	3	ProNova equipment. Founded by Scott Hamilton.
UTAH					
Huntsman Cancer Institute University of Utah 2000 Circle of Hope Salt Lake City, UT			801.585.0100 www.healthcare.utah.edu/ huntsmancancerinstitute/		Equipment to be determined.
VIRGINIA					
Inova Schar Cancer Institute at Inova Center for Personalized Health 3225 Gallows Road Fairfax, VA 22031		2G	571.472.2400 www.inova.org	2	Two IBA treatment rooms
WASHINGTON D.C.					
Johns Hopkins Sibley Hospital Proton Therapy Center 5255 Loughboro Rd NW, Washington, DC 20016	2019	3G 1F ?			2019
PROTON CENTERS CLOSED OR ON HOLD					
CALIFORNIA					
Los Angeles Country Proton Therapy Center 2822 Cabot Road Laguna Niguel CA 92677					Project was a scam. Developers were arrested. No construction ever started.

Name/Contact/Affiliation	Open	#Room	Contact Information	#PBS	Comments
Todd Cancer Pavillion Long Beach Memorial Medical Center 2810 Long Beach Boulevard Long Beach CA 90806					Seems to have been approved in 2013. No further action taken.
University of California at San Diego San Diego, CA					Decided to collaborate with other proton center in San Diego rather than competing.
Scripps Proton Therapy Center San Diego, CA					Went bankrupt in 2017. Now under new ownership as California Protons
ILLINOIS					
Northern Illinois University Decalb, IL					Abandoned due to lack of financing.
INDIANA					
Indiana University Proton Center Bloomington, IN					Decommissioned in 22014 due to antiquated equipment and poor management.
LOUISIANA					
Louisiana Proton Therapy Center New Orleans, LA					Provision lost its local partner. Development on hold.
MASSACHUSETTS					
Tufts University School of Medicine Boston, MA					Showed interest in 2012. No action in recent years.
TEXAS					
Dallas Proton Therapy Center Dallas, TX					Forced into bankruptcy due to shady dealing. Will not be built.

Share and Review

Right now my life's focus is on getting out the word about proton therapy. In virtually every conversation in which I bring up the subject, the other parties are unaware of proton therapy. Further, they all tell stories about a friend of a relative who had a very difficult time with their cancer treatment. If only they had known.

Even when someone tells me in great anguish that they have been diagnosed with cancer, my presentation of the potential of proton therapy often goes nowhere. They either forget, or dismiss it, or mention it to their doctor who warns against it.

It's a sad state of affairs that we must all work so hard to get proton therapy, and then work just as hard to have it covered by insurance. Now that you have read this book to the very end, I assume that you found this information useful. Please help to spread the word by telling others about this book (which also exists in ebook format). And, right now, while it is on your mind, go to Amazon.com and leave a positive review. If your response isn't positive, then please write me and express your opinion and suggestions directly (robert@ProtonTherapyBook.com). I want to get this right. You can help. Many thanks.

Robert D. Ferré
August, 2018

Preview

My second book about proton therapy covers many types of cancer, not just prostate cancer, including the following:

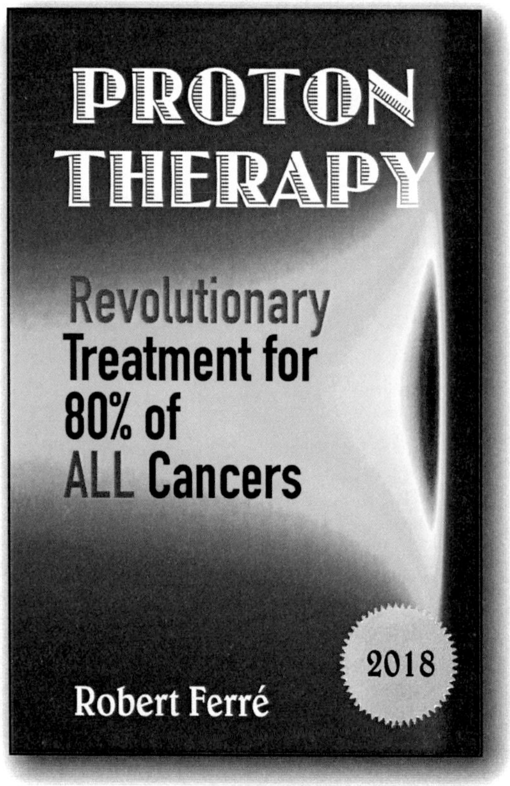

- Base of Scull
- Brain Tumors
- Breast Cancer
- Esophageal Cancer
- Head and Neck Cancer
- Hodgkin's Lymphoma
- Liver Cancer
- Lung Cancer (NSCLC)
- Optical Tumors
- Oropharynx Cancer
- Pancreatic
- Pediatric Cancers
- Pelvic Chondrosarcoma
- Prostate
- Recurrent
- Skin Cancer
- Spinal Cord Tumors

In all cases, the advantages of proton therapy are the same, namely, accuracy, sparing healthy tissue, and fewer side effects. Especially in the head, throat, and internal organs, protons can go where other treatments fear to tread. The prerequisite is that through some type of imaging, it must be possible to identify and locate the target. Just as proton therapy continues to improve, likewise so is imaging technology. We are all the beneficiaries.

There's a story behind the updating of my two books for 2018. In my original haste to get into print, I didn't properly get permission to use many of my illustrations. When those permissions were not forthcoming, I was obliged to make considerable changes to my books. I made them about twenty pages shorter and sell them only on Amazon. As a result, even though they are in full color, I was able to keep the price under twenty dollars. In fact, the retail price is only a dollar or so above the minimum price required by Amazon.

The proton therapy center in Prague, the Czech Republic, came to my rescue and provided some gorgeous illustrations comparing the results of X-rays to proton therapy. Here's an example for prostate cancer. Photons (on the left) are X-rays.

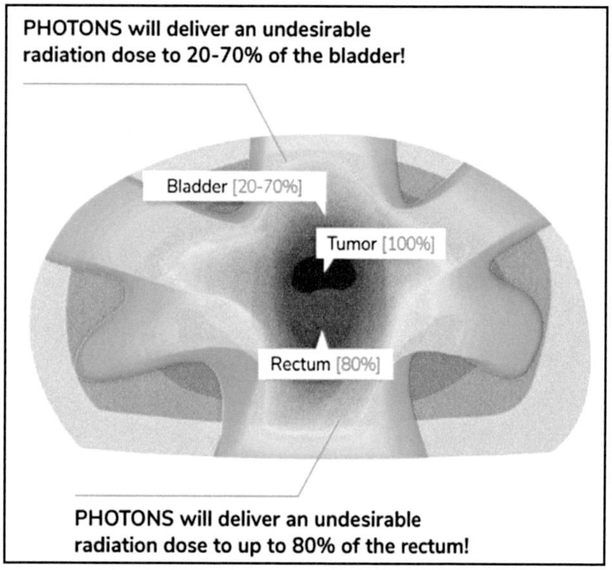

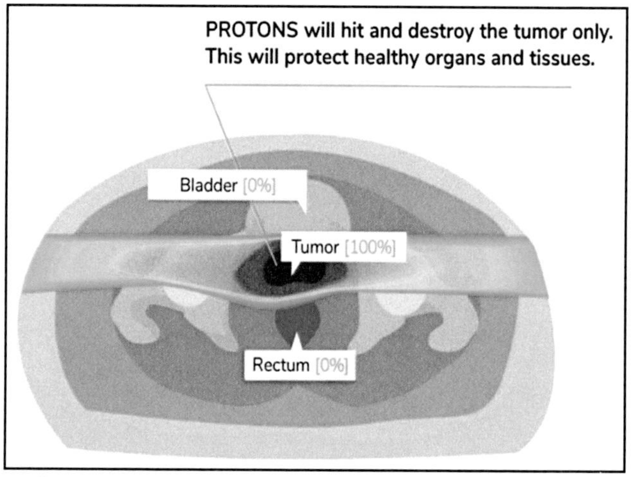

The print versions of my two books were followed by the ebook editions. Because some kindles are black and white only, I have put all of the illustrations from both books, plus some extras, on my website: www.ProtonTherapyBook.com. Previous versions of my books are no longer available. I have worked hard on these books and websites; now it's up to you, the reader, to pass on this information to anyone who is facing a cancer diagnosis. We can't count on their doctors to suggest it, so it's up to each of us to step in. I'm not suggesting giving medical advice, just drawing attention to this information and sources to consult. Doing so, we can save lives and prevent unnecessary suffering. It's a very high calling and responsibility, which I take seriously. I hope you will join me. Thanks.

NOTES:

90104517R00073

Made in the USA
San Bernardino, CA
06 October 2018